THE ALCOHOLIC FAMILY
IN RECOVERY

THE ALCOHOLIC FAMILY IN RECOVERY

A DEVELOPMENTAL MODEL

Stephanie Brown
Virginia Lewis

THE GUILFORD PRESS
New York   London

© 1999 The Guilford Press
A Division of Guilford Publications, Inc.
72 Spring Street, New York, NY 10012
www.guilford.com

Printed in the United States of America.

This book is printed on acid-free paper.

Last digit is print number: 9   8   7   6   5

Library of Congress Cataloging-in-Publication Data

Brown, Stephanie, 1944–
    The alcoholic family in recovery: a developmental model /
Stephanie Brown, Virginia Lewis.
        p.   cm.
    Includes bibliographical references and index.
    ISBN 1-57230-402-2 (hc.)   ISBN 1-57230-834-6 (pbk.)
    1. Recovering alcoholics—Family relationships. 2. Alcoholics—
Rehabilitation. 3. Temperance—Psychological aspects. 4. Family
psychotherapy. I. Lewis, Virginia (Virginia M.) II. Title.
HV5132.B748   1999
362.292'3—dc21   98-36077
                                                            CIP

For our research families,
with gratitude

About the Authors

Stephanie Brown, PhD, is a clinician, teacher, researcher, consultant, and author in the field of alcoholism. She founded the Alcohol Clinic at Stanford University Medical Center in 1977 and served as its director for 8 years, developing the dynamic model of alcoholism recovery and its application to the long-term treatment of adult children of alcoholics. Dr. Brown served on the California State Alcoholism Advisory Board and was a founding board member of the National Association for Children of Alcoholics. She is a recipient of the Bronze Key Award and the Humanitarian Award from the National Council on Alcoholism, the Community Services Award from the California Society for the Treatment of Alcoholism and Other Drug Dependencies, and an Academic Specialist Award from the USIA to teach in Poland. She will receive a Lifetime Achievement Award from the California Psychological Association in 1999. In addition to *The Alcoholic Family in Recovery*, Dr. Brown's other publications include *Treating the Alcoholic: A Developmental Model of Recovery* (Wiley, 1985), *Treating Adult Children of Alcoholics: A Developmental Perspective* (Wiley, 1988), *Adult Children of Alcoholics in Treatment* (coauthor, Health Communications, 1989), *Safe Passage: Recovery for Adult Children of Alcoholics* (Wiley, 1992), and *Treating Alcoholism* (editor, Jossey-Bass, 1995). She has also completed two training videos (Jaylen Productions). Dr. Brown is a licensed psychologist with 25 years of clinical experience. She is an internationally recognized expert on the trauma and the treatment of alcoholics and their families and is especially well known for her pioneering work in the theory and treatment of adult children of alcoholics. A Research Associate at the Mental Research Institute in Palo Alto, California, where she is Co-Director of the Family Recovery Project, Dr. Brown also maintains a private practice and directs the Addictions Institute in Menlo Park, California.

Virginia Lewis, PhD, is Co-Director of the Family Recovery Project and Senior Research Fellow at the Mental Research Institute in Palo Alto, California. In addition to her full-time private practice, she gives lectures and workshops on the Family Recovery Project and is coordinating and analyzing test data for journal publications. She has coauthored and been awarded several research grants with associates at the Mental Research Institute over the past 20 years, and has lent her skills to a number of research projects. She is a recipient of the Don D. Jackson Award for her development of the Family Goal Attainment Scale. Dr. Lewis has been in the field of psychology since the late 1960s. After spending many years providing psychological services, she returned to school to complete her doctorate in Clinical Psychology in 1986. She is a licensed psychologist, educational psychologist, and marriage, family, and child counselor. Dr. Lewis has taught many graduate courses in the field of clinical application and assessments, as well as chairing and serving as a committee member on a number of dissertation projects. She is coauthor, with Stephanie Brown, of "The Alcoholic Family: A Developmental Model of Recovery," a chapter appearing in *Treating Alcoholism* (Jossey-Bass, 1995). Dr. Lewis's current professional interests are expanding the family recovery typology model.

Acknowledgments

We started our Family Recovery Project at the Mental Research Institute (MRI), Palo Alto, California, in June 1989. Almost 10 years later, we present this book and we say thank you to countless individuals and institutions who helped us define a model of recovery for the alcoholic family.

Our research, from start to finish, has been a labor of love. When we began, few people grasped the idea of "family recovery." Yet, as we described our project, interest mounted. People all over the country offered their unbridled enthusiasm and concrete support. Step by step, one family at a time, our work came to fruition.

We thank our individual donors, Yale Jones, Eugenia Durdall, Rudy Driscoll, and an anonymous benefactor, who cheered us on and held us together financially. We are very grateful.

Lending their considerable experience in structured treatment programs, Ruth Anderson of El Camino Hospital and Barry Rosen of Sequoia Hospital joined us to explore and uncover the needs of families in recovery from the perspective of early abstinence. Their frontline input was invaluable. We also thank Jerry Moe of the Betty Ford Center for his early input in thinking about the design of a children's component.

As the word of our project spread, the volunteers called. We could not have undertaken this massive study without their help. We thank Lisa Abrams, Lois Allen-Byrd, Candace Atkins, Nora Kane, Makenzie Brown-Harris, Natalie Compagni, Shirley Goodfriend, Roger Greene,

Jeannette Johnson, Hal Linebarger, Jan Lyons, Patrick MacAfee, Patricia McCaffrey, Leslie Rivlin, and Joyce Schmid. We give extra thanks to Ben Hammett, who has contributed in countless ways over the entire life of the project.

We also thank our volunteer institutions: Merritt Peralta Institute, Summit Medical Center, and El Camino Hospital contributed space for field testing our educational program (MAPS) for families. Patrick MacAfee, Summit Medical Center, Serenity Lane, and MRI also contributed space for research interviews and testing.

We thank staff who have organized and managed the huge tasks of data collection, entry, and analysis. Orit Atzmon, Hagit Bachrach, Margo Chapin, George Graham, Virginia Logan, and Leslie O'Neill have given the research ongoing containment, form, and statistics, a monumental achievement in coping with more variables than we ever imagined.

We are deeply grateful to MRI for institutional support and generous consideration of our professional and personal needs. It has been wonderful to have a positive "home," with such enthusiastic support.

Our project has spawned many branches over these 9 years. We appreciate and thank Donna-Lloyd Kolkin and Lisa Hunter of Health and Education Communication Consultants for their vision of a video and CD–ROM component to our curriculum project.

We thank our growing group of dissertation students, including Diane Petroni, Gwen Marvin, and Bob Navarra, who have contributed so much to our knowledge base as they have built their own.

Most of all, we thank our 52 volunteer families and couples who offered to share their experiences of drinking and recovery with us. It was not a small gift. They spent 6 or more hours with us in the interview and testing and they opened themselves to unexpected feelings and insights. It was an emotional investment and a trust in the value of our work that was vital to us. We are deeply grateful.

Early on, we asked three recovering couples to meet with us once as a focus group to help us design the research. At the end of the 2-hour meeting, they said "more." All agreed they needed a forum to share their experiences as couples in recovery. We met together once a month for 5 years. We learned so much from them and both felt tremendously enriched by the process.

We thank Kitty Moore, our editor at The Guilford Press, for helping us with the very difficult task of translating research data into a clinically relevant and useful text. We also thank Judith Grauman, Editorial Supervisor of The Guilford Press, and Bert N. Zelman, of Publishers Workshop Inc., for their superb work.

It has been a long, hard road to get to our model and this book. Just like the process of recovery for the alcoholic family, we have progressed through stages, ups and downs, the threat of collapse, and the hope of survival. We made it, and we thank each other for the commitment, endurance, and trust in the process.

Individually, we also have thanks.

Stephanie: I am deeply grateful to my known and unknown (to me) friends, colleagues, patients, and members of AA and Al-Anon who have supported me and my work for over 25 years. I have been so blessed to know individuals and families who have been there, who have stopped drinking and changed dramatically, both in the short term and over the long haul. I have been challenged, surprised, and deeply moved by the families who shared their experiences with us in the Family Recovery Project. I thank them again.

I thank Virginia Lewis for her commitment to this wide-open, unknown territory and her wonderful management of all the pieces. Virginia's strengths in methodology and systems theory guided us throughout.

I also thank the staff of The Addictions Institute for their long-standing support of me and the developmental perspective of addiction. I look forward to the continuing challenge of bridging addiction and mental health theory and practice as we continue to teach, write, and work together.

Finally, always and ever, I can't do any of this without my family, my husband, Bob Harris, and our daughter, Makenzie. Again, I offer my enduring love and gratitude to them.

Virginia: Personally, this project could not have been undertaken without a strong homebase of friends and family. We both have other full-time professional commitments, so for me, homecoming was a continual gift of support, quietness, and renewal. At the same time, this research has been transformative in deep and frequently challenging ways because of all of those who gave so generously in time, spirit, and depth and wealth of information.

I am indebted to many and to two specifically, Stephanie Brown and Ben Hammett. To Stephanie for her passionate commitment to the research, her creative thinking, and her dynamism. To Ben for his profound dedication to this project—he was willing to undertake any task regardless of how big or how small with his quiet competence and willing smile.

I am continuing my involvement in the analysis of the family data for journal contributions and workshops. We have an enormous database of measures and have only begun to scratch the surface of understanding these dynamics of families in recovery in this project.

Preface

This is a book about recovery from alcoholism for the whole family. We talk about couples with no children, families with young children, and families with grown-up children.

In this book, we ask and answer one fundamental question: What happens to the entire family, as a system, when one or both parents stop drinking? As it turns out, the answer is not simple. A lot happens —a lot of change, on multiple levels, that is very positive, yet at the same time very difficult. We are going to describe the complicated process, including the ups and the downs, that families experience.

While many books have been written about the alcoholic, the coalcoholic (or codependent), and the children of alcoholics, nothing yet exists to describe the normal, natural process of recovery from addiction from the perspective of the whole family. That's what we're setting out to do here. We will map out a theory of short-term and long-term development and change, identifying the key stages and tasks for the family and the implications for the therapist.

WHAT WE DID

For more than 25 years, I (SB) have been asking the question: What is the normal process of recovery for the individual? After outlining the experiences of abstinence and stages in a long-term process of recovery for the alcoholic, the coalcoholic, and the children of alcoholics (Brown, 1985, 1988, 1991a, 1991b, 1991c, 1995a, 1995c), it was a natural next step to ask what happens to the family as a whole. Is there a "normal" developmental process of recovery for the family similar to the long-term process of change for the individual?

The answer is "yes," a resounding "yes." In this book we outline a model of family recovery based on the Family Recovery Project, a study we began in 1989 at the Mental Research Institute (MRI). We asked volunteer couples and families who defined themselves as "being in recovery" from alcoholism to tell us what happened to them, as individuals and as a family, when they were drinking and after they stopped (see Appendix A).

With a dedicated, largely volunteer staff, we completed the research at four sites, a geographic spread that helped us achieve an anonymous (to us) and varied sample. Through word of mouth and advertisements in local newspapers and newsletters, we recruited our participants.

In addition to anonymity, we hoped to achieve some measure of diversity, including gender, ethnicity, religious affiliation, and ongoing sources of support (including Alcoholics Anonymous, Al-Anon, Alateen, psychotherapy, and/or religious involvement). We were successful on all accounts except ethnicity. Although we advertised and attempted to directly recruit non-Caucasian volunteers, we only obtained a small number.

We hoped that families who identified themselves as "recovering" would be interested in this study and willing to participate. Those who did volunteer were, indeed, interested and willing (though some members of individual families were not), and we are very grateful to them. Many of our families wanted to give something back in gratitude for all they had been given. Others thought the research would help them with problems they were experiencing. Even though we asked for a huge time commitment—the research took about 6 hours—we, naively, did not anticipate as much resistance as we encountered. Despite pleas through various channels, we found it difficult to obtain as many subjects as we had hoped to have.

Although, as we note in our acknowledgments, the idea of "family recovery" generated enthusiasm and support, we also found that it was threatening to both professionals and families. Our results indicate why. The process is surprising, very difficult, and unpredictable in many ways. It is hard work to do what these families have done and it was hard for many of them to tell us about it—both what it was like then and what it's like now. All were deeply grateful for recovery and for the help they'd been given, though no one told us it had been easy.

Ironically, we had volunteers we could not accept, and they were not happy. A single mother told us we were missing the boat in defining "couple" as a two-person, heterosexual pair, and "family" as a two-person, heterosexual pair with children or stepchildren of any age. She told us it was important to learn about recovery for the single parent. We couldn't agree more.

We also agree with several gay/lesbian couples who wanted to volunteer and were disappointed in our limited protocol. We wish we could have included everyone. In our trials, we found too many intervening variables to be able to compare different kinds of couples and families. We hope other researchers will fill these holes.

FOR WHOM IS THIS BOOK INTENDED?

We have written this text primarily for therapists who work with individuals, couples, and families with alcoholism during drinking and during recovery. We think therapists will be surprised and perhaps resistant to our findings, because so much goes against common expectations of what change is or should be. Therapists may also feel relieved, because what we report is what they have seen. Recovery is not a short-term fix.

We have also written this book for families—both those who are still drinking and those who are in recovery—who we hope will find help and hope in the experiences we describe. We expect families to be less surprised than therapists, because the rugged road we outline will match their experiences. Yet they, too, may be resistant, especially if they want to solve the expected problems of recovery easily. This book is not sugar-coated. It is a testimony that stopping drinking and being engaged in a long-term process of change is worth it absolutely, but it isn't easy. So, we anticipate that therapists and families alike will approach this text with mixed feelings. There is no quick fix for anything.

WHAT IS THE FOCUS?

In this book, we confine our focus to the developmental model of recovery, outlining the stages of recovery, the domains of experience in recovery, and the key tasks for the family and the therapist at each stage. Because we rely heavily on verbatim quotations from our research families, we have changed identifying information extensively. In some instances, we have constructed composite families, without, we believe, altering the point of the quote or example.

While many of our families had been in therapy previously, and were in therapy (as well as 12-step recovery programs) at the time of the interview, our questions and the framework of the study were not clinical. We wanted to find out what happened to the family when the adult alcoholics stopped drinking. That is what we will present. We will also comment on the clinical meaning of this material throughout.

While the focus of the book is theory, we also emphasize clinical listening. How and what the therapist listens for and what the therapist hears are critical to every aspect of treatment. In our view, it is the developmental model that frames listening.

A word of warning: The reader will find repetition. The stages and the tasks of development are a layered, building-block process based on repetition, just like much of normal human development and change. We repeat the basics as the recovering families are repeating them. Here, we emphasize the importance of repetition to successful growth and development—for families and therapists.

WHAT'S AHEAD?

We have divided the book into four parts. In Part I, we outline key assumptions and definitions that formed a foundation for the research and the results. We spell out our biases in favor of abstinence, 12-step programs, the cornerstone experience of loss of control, and the developmental frame. We also highlight the principles of the developmental model, which we describe in greater detail throughout the text. Finally, we discuss assessment and the art of listening with alcohol addiction as an organizing focus.

In Part II, we present the stories of four families in recovery. We relate these narratives in detail to give the reader a clear sense of the families talking with us. We also add clinical comments to illustrate how we are listening and what we are hearing within the developmental frame. These families serve as examples for the theoretical material that follows.

In Part III, we define the domains of experience, including the environment, the family system, and individual development, with a focus on assessment of family function. Next, we summarize the stages of recovery for the family, including the primary tasks for the family and the therapist. Finally, we outline several differentiating factors that influence recovery.

In Part IV, we present the developmental model of recovery in detail. We devote a chapter to each stage, outlining the domains of experience and the task for the family, the couple, and the individuals—the alcoholic, the coalcoholic, and the children.

Finally, we present a glossary and appendices with data on the research sample.

We hope and expect that therapists from all schools will find that their solid clinical skills will readily carry over to work with recovering families. We offer the developmental model, and perhaps even the idea of family recovery, as the framework for determining clinical intervention.

Contents

PART IV. A DEVELOPMENTAL MODEL OF FAMILY RECOVERY

PART ONE

Introduction

CHAPTER ONE

What Happens When
the Drinking Stops?

This is a book about the alcoholic family in recovery. Why the family? Much of the literature on addiction and its treatment still focuses on the drinking alcoholic, with little or no attention to the family as a whole. In seminal works, Joan Jackson (1954, 1962) described the spouse of the alcoholic many years ago, and Steinglass, Bennett, Wolin, and Reiss (1987) outlined the dynamics of the alcoholic family more recently. But neither focused on recovery. And, as was true for the individual alcoholic, coalcoholic, and children of alcoholics 20 years ago, there is still no knowledge base about the family's experience of recovery. All of the attention has been on drinking, with the implication that abstinence would be the answer to everyone's problems. It was incorrectly believed that if the alcoholic stopped drinking and participated in a program of recovery (perhaps professional treatment and definitely Alcoholics Anonymous), the family would heal itself. Not so. We know from years of clinical experience and from the wealth of information now available regarding children of alcoholics that alcoholism affects the entire family, as individuals and as a whole. So does recovery. We wanted to find out how.

We already knew that many marriages and partnerships do not survive addiction. But what about recovery? Is the damage of drinking so great for some that, in their view, they are beyond repair? Or, is recovery itself so full of unexpected change that many couples give up,

3

determining that abstinence has *not* solved the family's problems after all, and there is no hope for the couple? Who stays together, why, and how do they do it?

As you'll hear from couples and families in recovery, abstinence is as hard or even harder than drinking because it reveals so many problems that were obscured by the family's focus on alcohol. Denial looms as large as ever as the family faces the harsh realities of delusion, illusion, and collusion that predominated during the drinking and that are now laid bare by abstinence. In so many families, the entire system became organized by alcoholism. What is left to organize the family in recovery?

With the knowledge that many couples end their relationships following abstinence, we wanted to know what happens for the couple that stays together. Why are they still together in recovery and how has this occurred? Have they had certain experiences, or completed tasks that have helped and what do they know about the pitfalls?

Is it possible that some couples end their relationships too soon (and others not soon enough) because recovery in the first few years is so hard, and because there is no "map" to chart the way and no other couples with whom to share their experiences? We believe this is so. Not every couple will or should survive recovery. But many more couples might decide to wait with a little more knowledge about what is normal based on the experience of those who have come before. In this book, you'll hear that many of our families are glad they waited; and some don't know yet.

THE RESEARCH

These questions formed the base of the Family Recovery Research Project. We worked with 52 couples and families with lengths of abstinence ranging from 79 days to 18 years. We asked them to participate in a live, 3-hour, audio- and videotaped interview, to take five tests of individual and family function, and to answer a comprehensive demographic questionnaire. In contrast to this one-time interview and testing, we also worked with three couples with long-term sobriety in an ongoing couples group. Meeting once a month for five years, this group gave us data about the process of recovery for the intact couple over time. Finally, we developed a curriculum for families in recovery. Called MAPS (for Maintaining Abstinence Programs), it consisted of 12 weekly meetings for couples and families with more than a year of abstinence. In these meetings, we outlined the process of recovery for the family, based on our belief that education about what to expect and what is normal following abstinence would be helpful. It was. Participants unanimously valued the information and the experience of sharing with other couples and families. The research interview is in Appendix A, and a summary of the study sample is in Appendix B.

A critical aspect of this research and prior studies involves membership in Alcoholics Anonymous (1955) and Al-Anon (1984). In the original study (Brown, 1985) of the individual alcoholic, all subjects were members of AA. Thus, the model that emerged was a theory of recovery only for people who stopped drinking *and* belonged to AA.

In our Family Recovery Research Project, membership in AA and Al-Anon was not required. It turned out that the majority of self-identified alcoholics did belong to AA and a smaller percentage of their partners belonged to Al-Anon (see Appendix B, Table B.1). A few of our couples used religion and/or therapy as their primary source of support and had no involvement in AA or Al-Anon. Some used all.

Many of the individuals who used both the 12-step recovery program and therapy viewed them as complementary. We heard few, if any, worries that therapy might interfere with the 12-step philosophy, a concern expressed by many of the participants in the research on alcoholics 20 years ago (Brown, 1985). In fact, many felt their 12-step recoveries were greatly enhanced by individual, couple, or family therapy.

We found that the developmental model describes a process of profound change over time, which is very much related to being in AA and Al-Anon but not limited to these programs. The critical mechanisms of change involved the experience of "hitting bottom," the acceptance of "loss of control," *and* reaching *outside* the family for help.

We found significant differences in the experience and the process of recovery depending on whether both partners, one partner, or neither sought outside help. To a very significant degree, the ability to seek help and engage with help outside the family was the most critical factor facilitating long-term change. We will emphasize this paradoxical finding throughout the book.

We state it now because we are very biased. We both believed in the positive benefits and, indeed, the power of AA and Al-Anon before we started, and this belief shaped our work. We still do. In this book, we will confirm "loss of control," the core of AA philosophy (Brown, 1985, 1993), as the central organizing principle of active addiction, abstinence as the cornerstone of recovery, and the un-equivocal value of AA and Al-Anon. We learned something about why these programs are so helpful to the individuals and the family, which we will report.

From our interviews with families, a theory emerged that is consis-tent with the earlier developmental model of recovery for the individual. We will outline what recovery is like, what to expect, and even what's normal. Abstinence marks the beginning of a new developmental process that has a profound, complicated impact on the whole family.

The theory that emerged from our research confirmed our clinical experience but also yielded unexpected findings. It sometimes shocked the families, and it may also surprise our readers. The necessary, normal process of growth and development goes against some cher-ished beliefs of what *should* be normal and healthy, and especially how we think people change. It also challenges therapists' principles and ideas about practice: what to do, what not to do.

This model of change is counterintuitive. It goes against the grain of what we tend to think is normal. So, some therapists may well have to shift figure and ground, letting go of *their* ideas of what change should look like and how it occurs; otherwise, what we describe below won't make sense. This turning upside down is exactly what families have to face as well.

It is never easy. In fact, many of our assumptions (based on Brown's prior research) in undertaking the work are still controversial among professionals. Certainly families who are still drinking fight these core principles, sometimes almost literally "to the death." Only from the vantage point of being "in recovery" can they see that their old beliefs, behaviors, and conflicts kept them drinking and kept them locked in pathology. Let us now look at the controversial assumptions and paradoxes that underlie and shape the whole book.

KEY ASSUMPTIONS AND PARADOXES

1. *Abstinence is not recovery.* Abstinence provides a necessary foundation for the beginning of a developmental process of recov-

ery. With the cornerstone of abstinence in place, the entire family may embark on a major process of change that occurs both quickly and slowly over time.

2. *Recovery is a developmental process, not a singular event and not a prescribed outcome.* Becoming abstinent is a process and an event. It is also an outcome—the targeted goal of treatment interventions. Today, since many therapists are strictly problem focused, help can mean fixing people and a belief that therapeutic success should come quickly, with measurable improvements. While a focus on problem resolution can be enormously useful for many kinds of difficulties, it can severely limit the therapist who is working with the drinking or recovering alcoholic family.

With our emphasis on process, we're talking about the big picture, the long haul, and a natural order of change. Time is essential. Much of the process is evolutionary and developmental, rather than prescriptive. Change is incremental and layered. It builds on itself. It is also a process of "fits and starts," as one family described it:

> "We went through a series of crises which pushed us to a new level. Then we'd stabilize until another crisis would push us again."

As an interactive process individuals must accommodate to the changes they are making, which in turn generate further change and accommodation. Several of our families described this process as a "ripple" effect. Change builds upon itself and leads to other changes.

A couple with 8 years of recovery illustrates:

> "The kinds of changes we were making at 5 years simply weren't possible at 6 months, nor did they have the same meaning. Change is the result of the accumulated strengths of the new foundation. The positive energy of recovery gave us different attitudes, which changed the way we related to each other."

Still, therapists will ask: What kind of success is it when many people feel worse, look worse, and function worse in abstinence than they did when they were drinking? And what kind of outcome is this if everyone is happy about it, or at least philosophical and accepting? What kind of outcome is it if the family says that it's falling apart, that nothing works anymore, nothing makes any sense, and they're all grateful they got here—or that it's so bad they don't know if it's worth it or whether they should stay together? Many therapists, looking for measurable improvement, will not have an easy time with such outcomes, at least at first.

In a developmental frame, human beings are dynamic, fluid, and changing, rather than static. So are families. Applied to alcoholism and the alcoholic, abstinence is not an end or a static state but the beginning of a new process of development.

In the developmental view, growth and change occur over time and can be defined according to the particular task and stage. Growth is hierarchical in the sense that the early or beginning tasks and stages lay a foundation on which further, more complex development can occur. Problems in the successful completion of any task or stage may be traced to unfinished tasks or missing pieces along the way. Holes in development can contribute to ongoing problems that require intervention and repair.

The developmental view applies to most theories of human growth ranging from the biological (including neurological and psychophysiological) to cognitive, behavioral, and emotional approaches. It also applies to the progression of drinking and recovery. The program of AA, including the 12 steps, outlines a *process* of growth that takes place over time in which each task and stage follows from and builds on the preceding one.

Through "working the program" individuals in AA and Al-Anon learn how to track their ongoing development in recovery, including watching for problems and recognizing holes that need attention and perhaps repair. Many individuals and families in therapy are doing the same thing.

In this longer, comprehensive view, what might be labeled as a problem—to be fixed—in a short-term frame, can be seen instead as part of a stage, part of a process. It may seem and, in fact, it may be very negative in the up-close moment, but a wide-angle lens casts a different view. It gives context and perspective. We may then decide whether or not to intervene. We do not assume the family is headed in the wrong direction, although we assess the possibility. It is just as likely that they are actually moving toward a more positive way of relating. We might tell them, for example, that the disruption and turmoil they are experiencing at 6 weeks' or 3 months' abstinence is normal, that they do not need to try to stop it, or fix it. Families do need support in living with it, however, which we would address directly. Are they going to meetings, sharing with others? At this point in time, we assess structural support rather than targeting symptom reduction as the goal.

What does this mean for therapists? Being in recovery is not itself a problem to be treated, though unfortunately it is sometimes seen this way. That's because recovery is often just as traumatic as drinking, but in different, paradoxical ways. Many changes that are necessary to move to abstinence and to set a recovery foundation in place are themselves traumatic. Thus, individuals and families are faced with the dilemma that what is absolutely necessary to establish and maintain recovery can *also* cause problems and even damage, without awareness and support. Years into recovery, families may go back to remember and resolve the trauma of "what it was like" and "what happened" in drinking *and* recovery.

Being in recovery is a normal process, with clearly defined, predictable tasks and stages. It is absolutely vital for therapists to know what is normal over time in the process of recovery or they may inadvertently try to treat, stop, or fix what is normal and necessary to growth. It is the therapist's job to stay out of the way of the natural healing process, to monitor progress, and to recognize past or current roadblocks that might interfere with people's ability to remain abstinent and engaged in recovery. It is also the therapist's job to know the path, to anticipate the seemingly unresolvable conflicts families will face, and to help them cope with these challenges in ways that will minimize secondary trauma. The complicated task for the therapist is to constantly assess what is part of growth—for this person and this family—and what is a sign of difficulty that requires intervention. The individuals and the family hopefully are doing the same thing.

It is the therapist's task to listen, interpret, advise, educate, and coach all along the way. It is not the therapist's job to dictate what change should be. For example, the therapist is not approaching the family with a goal of helping people express their feelings more or less, based on the therapist's idea of what constitutes good therapy. The therapist instead wonders how the expression of feeling *at this point in time*, in this particular family, will facilitate or inhibit the developmental process of recovery. The therapist is always guided by a focus on the organizing principles of loss of control, abstinence, and the long-term, developmental process.

3. *Recovery is an interaction and an interactive process, meaning that there is no predetermined end or goal to achieve.* It's an interaction of the individual's relationship to self and other and family members' relationships with one another. It's an interaction that builds on itself,

reinforcing and strengthening the foundation that will hold and later shape healthy couple and family relationships. Recovery is the result of the individuals' and couples' participation in it.

4. *This interaction creates a constant, what some might even call a chronic, tension within the family: the tension between the focus on the individuals and the focus on the family as a whole.* Both are vital, though the primary focus changes depending on the particular stage and task at hand. In the beginning, confusion about what is necessary and what is desirable often causes serious difficulties.

Couples need to tolerate ongoing ambiguity as part of this tension. They need to tolerate not knowing much about anything, which is often so frightening it pushes people to premature action and closure. Recovery in the beginning is so new and so shocking, and reality is so different from everyone's dream, that it is sometimes hard to find a basis for hope. It is also hard to trust in the natural process and to follow a path, usually AA and Al-Anon, when the impulse is to seize control, carve out one's own plan, and end the state of "not knowing" and uncertainty.

This is why it is essential for therapists to know what is normal over a long period of time. They can help the couple and family tolerate all the unknowns by literally mapping out the terrain, offering support and suggestions for coping, as well as tracking progress and pitfalls.

5. *AA, Al-Anon, and other 12-step programs are valuable sources of help for people who are facing addiction.* Unlike most professional therapies, the "message" of recovery is carried through an apprentice model. That is, people who have come before share their "experience, strength and hope" with those who are following (Alcoholics Anonymous, 1955). Through this supportive, reassuring chain of shared experience, individuals learn how to maintain abstinence and build sobriety. We will emphasize and illustrate how membership in a 12-step program helps people tolerate all the tension, ambiguity, and "not knowing," and literally "holds" (Winnicott, 1953) the family through the recovery trauma of massive disruption, change, and new development.

6. *Therapists can also be valuable sources of help for people who are facing addiction.* In tracking the normal process of recovery, therapists will stand ready to intervene at behavioral, cognitive, psychodynamic, and systems levels, based on the stage and task of recovery and the needs of *this particular family.* As noted above, intervention is guided by a focus on maintaining abstinence and the organizing principles of

the developmental model, particularly loss of control. It is not determined by a therapist's preferred treatment modality, a shift in frame that is often difficult for therapists. Having been trained to specialize in one school—behavioral, cognitive, psychodynamic, or systems— therapists may impose their preferred approach on all patients, expecting them to fit. In many cases, because of a too-specialized, limited theoretical frame and a focus on problem resolution, the therapist ends up ignoring the patient's experience and the known stages and tasks of recovery. Many therapists are as impatient as the family to finish up with this nasty business of addiction and get on with the "real work." Nothing could be more off base.

Frequently, therapists believe that recovery, or change, comes from the therapist rather than the patient. Much of experimental research and some theories of change rest on these premises: what can the therapist *do* to a patient, or what "intervention" can the therapist bring that will *cause* the patient to change? This thinking can increase the danger that the therapist will fall into the exact "thinking disorder" that the alcoholic is struggling with: the therapist assumes the faulty belief that he or she is the agent of change and is thus responsible for figuring out how to *get* the patient to stop drinking. In essence, therapists get caught in the faulty belief that they must control the patient, the same distorted logic of the alcoholic and family. If there's a problem, someone else is responsible for solving it. The same kind of distortion occurs in recovery. Everyone, including the therapist, wants to fix this disaster as soon as possible. Accepting that it can't be fixed and, in fact, that all is going well is very difficult.

While directed interventions are frequently helpful, therapists must accept their own limitations in being able to *make* anybody change. This truism is often a major source of countertransference: therapists have as much distaste for the idea and reality of "loss of control" as the patients they are treating.

As in any other clinical work, therapist beliefs can be a major source of help and hindrance. For example, therapists may feel frustrated when alcoholism is identified and yet the family rejects the whole idea. The therapist expects everyone to go along with abstinence. Or the therapist and family may agree to behavior changes that will support abstinence, but no one looks at the family's beliefs about alcoholism. Later, after several relapses and great family resistance to change, it becomes clear that no one in the family wants Mom to be an alcoholic and they don't want to be an "alcoholic family." The failure to explore the family's beliefs, values, and wishes interferes with behavioral change. The therapist, having grown up with an alcoholic father, unconsciously supported the resistance. He or she didn't want to be part of an alcoholic family either. Finally, another therapist may see that "good psychotherapy" involves a focus on the transferential relationship between the patient and the therapist. This clinician sees the newly abstinent patient's attention to concrete behavioral change and intense engagement in AA as resistance to engagement in the therapeutic dyad and pushes the patient to focus more on the therapist, transference, and uncovering psychotherapy. The patient may respond in any of several ways: she or he complies but feels more conflict; or the patient ends the therapy; or the patient drinks. These examples characterize the ongoing challenge for the therapist: how to integrate complex mental health theories of psychotherapy and change with addiction knowledge. As we outline the stages and tasks of therapy for the alcoholic family, we will also comment on the difficult task for the therapist.

7. *The model of recovery is transformational* (Tiebout, 1944, 1946, 1949, 1953). Individuals who belong to 12-step programs speak about conversion, about surrender, and giving up, which involve a radical rupture in deepest belief—there is no alcoholism in this family and no one has lost control—followed by a starting-from-scratch process of development organized by the opposite belief—there is alcoholism in this family and everyone has lost control. The alcoholic has lost control of drinking, the partner cannot control the alcoholic, and everyone has lost control to the power of a drinking, pathological family system. Within this system, everyone's best efforts to "fix" the problem reinforce it. The transformation process involves two separate experiences: the individual(s) accept the loss of control *and* reach outside the family for help.

8. *The developmental model of addiction and recovery is organized by core beliefs about control.* Drinking is maintained by a false belief in control; recovery is organized by the deep acceptance of loss of control. As therapists working with drinking families, we are not trying to plug holes or help families regain control. We work to help them widen the holes so the defensive structure, based on the faulty belief in control, can collapse and the new building process of recovery begin. This is an ongoing dilemma for the therapist: how to facilitate increasing disruption knowing that the result will not be a "fixed" family. In most cases, individuals and families will feel worse and look worse. This goes directly against the grain of what many patients, therapists, insurers, and employers think ought to happen.

Individuals and families "in recovery" have undertaken what some might call a bone-breaking process of change. This is a radical shift in paradigm, not an adjustment or fine-tuning within the same organizing structure of belief. That is why it is transformational and counterintuitive. According to family systems theorists, the recovering family has made a shift from first- to second-order change (personal communication from V. Lewis to S. Brown, 1997).

9. *Recovery takes time*. There is nothing about recovery that is brief, or a quick fix. It is tough but necessary to relinquish the hope for a magical "fix" because the notion of a short-term cure is antithetical to the slower, healing-building process of recovery. Family members often struggle with this reality as they continue to hold onto the belief that the family's problems were caused by the drinking (and therefore by the alcoholic alone) and should be solved by abstinence (and therefore by the alcoholic alone). As long as abstinence is seen as the end of the problem, which is convenient for all, rather than the beginning of a new growth process that can involve all, the myth will continue: recovery should bring a reversal of trauma and much improved family function and relationship in a very brief period of time. All of these changes do occur, but not quickly. There is more disruption and turmoil that comes first—what we call the "trauma of recovery."

KEY DEFINITIONS

One of the most controversial areas of theory and practice in treating the alcoholic and the family is that of definitions. We will define some of the most critical terms and concepts here. A more detailed glossary is at the end of this book.

1. *What is alcoholism?* We define alcoholism as a physical, psychological, social, emotional, and spiritual disease, characterized by continuous or periodic loss of control of drinking, preoccupation with the drug alcohol, use of alcohol despite adverse consequences, and distortions in thinking, particularly denial. Although there has always been controversy about whether or not alcoholism is a disease (Marlatt, 1983; Pendery, Maltzman, & West, 1982; Jellinek, 1960), there is less disagreement that the term "alcoholism" denotes "loss of control." Abstinence is essential. Other schools of opinion do not use this term, preferring instead "problem drinking" and the currently popular "substance abuse." Both of these terms hold the possibility that control has

not been lost or that it can be regained. In our model, we use the term alcoholism (or addiction, to include drugs besides alcohol), the organizing principle of "loss of control," and the requirement of abstinence in order to qualify as a "family in recovery."

2. *What is recovery?* "Recovery" is now a common term, popularized by the chemical dependency field in the 1980s and long associated with AA literature. Despite its common usage, it's a complex term that actually has multiple meanings. Although we too will use the word "recovery" in this text, the dictionary definition is not what we mean.

In *Webster's* view (1961/1981), to recover means "to get or win back; . . . to bring oneself back to normal balance." In the case of the individual alcoholic, the term "recovery" has long implied a "return" to health, sanity, and well-being that presumably existed before the individual became alcoholic. In this sense, recovery is seen as a "restoration" of something lost.

This may be true for some—take away alcohol and indeed people are better and "restored." But for most, recovery is a new process of development. It involves not restoration of a prior state but dramatic changes over a long period of time that will lead to new health and well-being. Recovery has thus come to mean growth and fundamental change rather than restoration or going back; the word in this sense implies not just a "correction" within the same system, or paradigm, but an alteration of the fundamental worldview. The changes we are going to report involve a radical transformation, with a new paradigm, forming the foundation for a new developmental process.

3. *What is an alcoholic family?* An alcoholic family refers to a family in which the environment or context of daily life becomes dominated by the anxieties, tensions, and chronic trauma of active alcoholism. Alcohol, or someone's drinking, becomes the central organizing principle of the family system, controlling and dictating core family beliefs and influencing all aspects of behavior as well as cognitive and affective development.

There is considerable dissonance in the alcoholic family. What is often most visible and problematic, the alcoholism, is most vehemently denied. The denial operates to say to the world, "This doesn't happen here. This doesn't exist." Members of the family are engaged in a continuing crusade to make the alcoholic well or to simply enable the family to survive despite what is really happening. They are coping, trying to hold things together. When the consequences of the alcoholism become more visible and difficult to resolve (illness, job loss, physical abuse, and drunk driving arrests), the need for secrecy grows and the family becomes a closed system, cutting itself off from other sources of input and help.

Individuals within the family develop the same behavioral and thinking disorders as the alcoholic: they are controlled by the reality of alcoholism, and they must deny it at the same time. Individual development may be sacrificed to the greater needs of the unhealthy drinking family system.

4. *What is an alcoholic family in recovery?* The recovering alcoholic family is one in which one or both parents has stopped drinking and the family, as a whole or in parts, is actively engaged in a process of growth and change. Our research families identified themselves as "recovering families" in very different ways. But most agreed that "recovery" and "being in recovery" from alcoholism organized to a greater or lesser degree their identity as a family and the process of change.

Families with long-term abstinence speak about recovery as a process. They have a backward lens, a view of life since drinking that is a history, a story of change. Families with shorter-term abstinence do not yet have the perspective of time away from alcohol and often have no story of change except the new unknown state of abstinence. We will describe both.

5. *What is pathology?* When we use this word, we are referring to the defensive accommodations people make to adjust to and maintain active alcoholism. These defenses may mask other serious emotional problems, and/or they become the problems that drive people to seek help. Often, in a clinical setting, what we will work to define as unhealthy, or pathological, also represents the family's best efforts to cope with the reality that must be denied. In recovery, pathology may include the underlying problems that were masked by alcohol as well as the consequences of drinking and the family's adjustments to maintaining it. In a general way, we define pathology as the behavioral, cognitive, and affective processes that defensively narrow one's internal and external view of self and the world. Recovery involves an expansion in these capacities (Brown, 1988).

Let's look next at the major conclusions we drew from this research.

CHAPTER TWO

The Developmental
Process of Recovery

W̲hat we have learned about the normal developmental process of recovery for the family is surprising and yet not surprising at all, complicated and yet not so complicated, if you just stop and think about it. Once you're there, it's common sense, but it's not common sense at all when you're not there, when you're not past it and you don't have the advantage of a long backward glance to see that it all fits together and makes sense. This is, of course, what we tell our families in recovery—our research participants and our patients. It's what we tell therapists too. We're going to spell out our major findings now so that they do not get lost in the details and variability we will turn to shortly: the stories of families in recovery, or the particular focus or task within a domain or stage. These findings, which underlie the principles of the developmental model, inform therapeutic understanding and intervention at any point in time. These principles constitute the ordering schema of the new process of becoming abstinent and subsequent recovery. How family members hold these multiple, often conflictual, schematic levels affects their process of recovery. The ways in which the therapist holds and interprets these multiple levels also affects how he or she listens to, thinks about, and interprets what is happening in this family.

In the mid-1970s I (Brown, 1985) identified four stages in a long-term process of recovery for the individual alcoholic, namely, Drinking, Transition, Early Recovery, and Ongoing Recovery. I initially thought each stage was related to the time away from drinking, or length of abstinence. Yet it turned out that the different stages were defined much more clearly by task—what needed to happen—than time. It was clear that time away from drinking was very important, but the length of time in abstinence alone did not necessarily equal growth and change. In order for people to truly change, they need to be able to take action, to become engaged and be open to learn.

As a developmental process, recovery for the individual alcoholic who belongs to AA moves from the concrete act of stopping drinking to an understanding of "being alcoholic," to the opening up of feelings and honest, more meaningful self-exploration. At the foundation of the whole process of change is the deep acceptance by the individual that he or she has lost control of drinking and has accepted the identity of an "alcoholic." The individual, accepting these truths, reaches outside the self and asks for help, which sets the developmental process of recovery in motion. We asked, "How does this model apply to the family?"

PRINCIPLES OF THE DEVELOPMENTAL MODEL FOR THE FAMILY

1. The four stages—Drinking, Transition, Early Recovery, and Ongoing Recovery—are generalizable from the individual to the family. However, the tasks and focus are more complex for the family. We needed a structure that would include multiple factors and perspectives simultaneously: the individual and the individual in relation to others—the family system. Further, we knew from research about children of alcoholics that we needed to separate the experience and the impact of the environment, the context of life, from the workings of the system.

The process of recovery for the family unfolds developmentally along two separate but interactive tracks, the "domains" and the "stages" (see Figure 2.1). The "domains" focus on three arenas of change. These include the environment, the family system, and the individual. Changes occur simultaneously within these domains according to "Stage" of recovery. The stages are defined by the task of change and, loosely, by the length of time in abstinence.

2. Our work confirms early findings (Brown, 1986, 1988, 1991c, 1995c; Black, 1981; Wegsheider, 1981) that the environment, or

FIGURE 2.1. A developmental model of recovery for the family.

Drinking	Transition	Early Recovery	Ongoing Recovery
Environment			
System			
Individual Development			

context, of the drinking family is traumatic and very harmful to children and adults. The unsafe, potentially out-of-control environment continues as the context for family life into the Transition and Early Recovery stages, which may last as long as 3–5 years.

3. Our work also confirms that the system of the drinking family is restrictive, rigid, and closed (Steinglass et al., 1987; Brown, 1985). Preservation of this unhealthy system supersedes any healthy development of the individuals within it. As a corollary, adaptation to the unhealthy system also produces pathology.

The dominance of systems pathology is critical. Individual, couple, and family problems are often caused by the family's best efforts to cope with the realities of alcoholism. The family's defensive strategies to preserve attachments, unity, and stability end up causing more trauma, developmental arrest, and psychopathology. It is the adaptation to a traumatic environment, unhealthy systems dynamics, and unhealthy attachments that creates further disturbance.

4. In recovery, this unhealthy family system must collapse. That is, the defensive structures that maintain the pathology of the entire family must change. This may take the form of either a literal "collapse" or a slower erosion over time. The challenge to the airtight system permits attention to shift to the individuals and their develop-

ment in recovery. We will illustrate how differences in "degree" of collapse have an impact on the process of recovery. Again, this process is counterintuitive. Recovery is not "pulling the family together." It is "letting go"—letting the family system collapse. This "giving up" is often calamitous.

This finding—the need for family systems collapse—is central to our whole theory of recovery. It is the collapse of the family structures and defense mechanisms that protected and maintained the drinking that clears the ground for the transformative process of recovery. As one family said, "You're not just putting your life back together; it's a new life."

Yet most families and many professionals view this collapse as a failure or as an unfortunate by-product of the move to abstinence that should be corrected as soon as possible. Again, many families feel "stranded with abstinence" and want to "put the family back together again" quickly. It is difficult to see that problems arising in abstinence (e.g., a child is acting out) are occurring precisely *because* the family is "in recovery," and they need to be interpreted in this context. Viewed superficially, it is understandable that therapists and families would want to focus on restabilizing the system immediately. It is very difficult, however, to work toward destabilizing the drinking system and to maintain a destabilized system in recovery when this systems vacuum actually causes new problems. In fact, it is the collapse of the system from inside that is crucial to recovery. Reaching outside the family and relying on external sources of support (treatment programs, 12-step groups, therapists, religious affiliation) ironically offers the necessary stabilization. It's just not the kind of help that people want or think they need. Seeking outside help, especially AA and Al-Anon, facilitates the collapse of an unhealthy system.

Most people resist reaching out, preferring instead to keep their problems inside the family and trying to solve them from within. One family told us,

> "What we have is *a result* of building a new foundation, which we could not do from within the family. We had to reach outside in order to give up the old and change." (Emphasis added.)

One of the most important truths about couple and family recovery that we have learned is that this closing in, "not airing dirty linen," doesn't work. The family will continue to try to solve problems with the very methods that keep the problems going. Reaching outside the family is the best step toward change that any individual, couple, or family can make. Yet, it is also one of the hardest.

It is hard for individuals to understand that the couple can be "on hold" during the early period and that the growth that takes place for each individual will give them a new foundation on which to build a healthier couple relationship later. To turn attention so dramatically away from the couple in order to focus on individual recoveries takes faith. Jenny Adams, married 11 years to Marlon, who has 4 years of abstinence, illustrates:

> "In the beginning, if the couple is going to stay together, they need to know that there's a period of time when you coexist and you're not a couple. You may have parallel lives, you may even sleep in the same bed, but it's not a relationship per say. I think often women enter recovery with their husbands and think, 'Now I'll get my knight in shining armor.' We're not going to be saved just because the mate gets sober. So, if I had anything to say to other families . . . it's not that you're not a family, but there's coexistence, parallel lives, and that's OK."

At the end of drinking, couples most likely will be in crisis, probably disturbed in most aspects of their relationship. Often anger and hostility permeate what is left of the couple bond. Such a couple goes on hold in Transition, because each partner needs to set a foundation of individual recovery and they both are not yet competent to work on their relationship. They are simply too "young" in recovery and therefore incapable of bringing a mature, autonomous "self" to a couple partnership. An intense focus on the couple, prompted by an instinct to repair the relationship and promote "intimacy," will likely lead them back to the pathological dynamics of the drinking system. Sometimes this will also lead to relapse, particularly if the individual focus is sacrificed completely.

This is an example of the counterintuitive process of change (Haley, 1973). It is a common mistake for the therapist and couple to focus on visible signs of improvement and thus to see this natural holding time as a problem to be fixed.

Other couples are not in such crisis, nor do they see themselves as disturbed. One partner's entry into recovery may be the crisis that disrupts what both believed was a close, even happy bond. They constructed a balanced, workable couple relationship that included active alcoholism. With abstinence, both partners may feel a loss of closeness along with the loss of couple focus. They too are not competent to emphasize intimacy early on, though they may be strongly motivated to give up the separation and differentiation dictated by abstinence and membership in 12-step programs.

One of our couples, abstinent for 6 years with support from church and therapy, said they felt a great loss with recovery. Evan told us he was depressed and virtually silent for several years. Beth said she believed she'd never have him again. He was simply gone: dry, mute, and very sad.

We will be emphasizing throughout this book why it is so important to let the family system remain in a collapsed state, how families accomplish this, and how therapists can help. Without outside supports, and reassurance that this collapse and turmoil are normal, couples will likely interpret the ongoing disruption, uncertainty, and lack of couple focus as proof of their basic incompatibility and the failure of recovery to give them intimacy.

At this point, it is all counterintuitive. One of the "hidden truths" we will unearth and emphasize throughout the book is that the couple "breaks up" and stays "separated"—emotionally—for a long time into recovery, as described by Jenny above. It is this separation and the shift from a focus on the couple and family system to their own individual development that gives the couple a healthy foundation on which to build a new, stronger couple bond. But this takes a long time; so long that some don't make it to the other side. This "break up" is what Bader and Pearson (1988) call "differentiation" in their model of normal couple development. Individual attachment to 12-step programs interrupts and destabilizes symbiotic, hostile–dependent, or chaotic couple dynamics. This emotional "separation," with the development of individual autonomy, is essential to the long-term health of the couple. Unfortunately, partners rarely can recognize that such separation is a foundational building block of mature intimacy.

5. With the collapse of the unhealthy family system, the adults turn their attention to their own development, beginning a process of individual recovery, the third "domain." This new developmental process takes years, not days or months, and ultimately enables lasting, in-depth change within the family. This attention to the individuals ideally involves all members of the family.

Healthy individual development is sacrificed in alcoholic families. Adults become arrested in their life cycle processes and development, as they "turn toward" (Brown, 1985, 1988) adaptation to the pathology of alcoholism and the unhealthy system. They must repair the damage that resulted from their sacrifice of self and their attachment and adaptation to pathology. Usually, the focus on individual growth and change goes back further and deeper than the consequences of alcoholism. Many adults recognize that their individual recoveries involve a completely new process of growth, not just a repair.

The normal tasks of childhood development will be skewed toward accommodation to the dominance of unhealthy parents and the preservation of the drinking system. Children will grow up with significant internal and interpersonal problems that serve as their model for adult relationships and family life. The replication and repetition of pathology from one generation to the next is, without intervention and change, automatic (Brown, 1988, 1991a, 1991b, 1991c, 1995c; Black, 1981; Cermak, 1986).

Alcoholism has been called a "family generational" disease because it is passed on. In our sample, most of the adult alcoholics and their spouses had grown up with an alcoholic parent (they are referred to as ACOAs, or adult children of alcoholics), and many had alcoholic children. It was not unusual to have at least three generations of alcoholics identified. Many of the ACOAs had intense, unresolved childhood issues to contend with as well as their own adult recoveries. For many, alcoholism is more than a disease, more than a "part" of life. It is a legacy, a heritage, and a family identity.

These issues highlight the complexity of assessment and treatment and illustrate why it's helpful for the therapist to have a theoretical background in child and family development (Erikson, 1963; Mahler, Pine, & Bergman, 1975; Stern, 1985; Piaget, 1954, 1970; Flavell, 1963; Kagan, 1984; Bowlby, 1988; Blos, 1962; Sullivan, 1953) as well as addiction. For example, we see that past a critical age of about 10–12 years, children may resist joining the new family process. Already beginning the adolescent task of separation from the family, they are suddenly threatened by everything: the collapse of a system that they need in place, abstinence, and the pull to join the new emphasis on recovery. The adolescent needs a stable family to separate from. Recovery throws the unhealthy stability of the drinking system into new chaos. Not infrequently, children will act out immediately. In several of our families, adolescents began drinking and using other drugs in an out-of-control manner in direct response to a parent's abstinence.

6. Unfortunately, we learned that children may be just as neglected and abandoned in recovery as they were during the drinking, or more so, as the system collapses and parents turn their attention away from family onto themselves. From the perspective of the children, it may very well look and feel worse: the parents are as self-absorbed in recovery as they were dominated by the disturbed dynamics of the drinking family.

This was a shocking, disturbing finding: what is most important and necessary for the parents—the collapse of the couple system, reaching outside the family for help, and a shift to the individual focus—can be harmful to the children. It is not abstinence but the absence of the parents, who have reached outside the family, and their failure to watch out for the best interests of the children that causes the harm, just as it did during the drinking.

This dilemma of different needs contributes to chronic tension and conflict about what and who should be most important. It is not "all or none," though it often feels that way. With the collapse of the system and parents told to focus on themselves, kids will end up most acutely vulnerable. Who is watching out for them? They are often too young to be in charge of themselves and their own development. Yet, of course, this is what many have already known during the drinking. No one was in charge then either. But in recovery, it is difficult to be a child with needs when parents are told to go to meetings and to focus on themselves and sobriety. We heard from several families that they were told not to worry about their children, or to leave them home alone when they were much too young. A father told us, "I will be forever grateful for my wife's sobriety, but I live with guilt and regret that we abandoned our son in the early years to focus on ourselves."

In this book, we will be watching out for parents *and* children, acknowledging the realities and difficulties of being in recovery, and offering suggestions for building supports and structures so that children will not be harmed by the parents' focus on themselves. We will not take an either–or position: that the parents must not go to meetings or focus on their own programs of recovery because they must focus on their children *instead*; or, vice versa, that parents should forget about their children in the interests of their sobriety. It simply must not be all or none.

We will advocate the necessity of attending to both—parents *must* pay close attention to their individual recoveries *and* they must pay close attention to their children—while recognizing how very difficult this "double focus" can be. The problem of "attention" to self and/or other is a central issue for most couples and families, and a critical question in the culture today. Being suddenly "in recovery" gives these issues emergency status. We do not for a moment believe that the well-being of children should be ignored or sacrificed to the needs of their parents. We cannot prevent the trauma of all the change that comes with recovery, but we can help families add supports that will reduce the turmoil and the conflict that are consequences of the radical move to abstinence. Our work highlights in bold type the difficulty of relying only on oneself and believing that individuals and families must carry the burden of change alone. This is a book about the power of reaching outside the self and the family and relying on external sources of help. Of course, many will recognize this construct in its AA, Al-Anon context as the greater power of the group, and ultimately the "Higher Power" (Alcoholics Anonymous, 1955; Brown, 1993; Fowler, 1993). We advocate the spiritual dynamic of reliance on something greater than the self as a model to be translated into therapeutic interventions and the concept of extended, community support systems, an idea whose time has come culturally. We suggest that families in recovery can be "mentor" families to others, offering education and support in the tradition of the AA and Al-Anon sponsors.

7. Families are in a dynamic process of difficult change for as long as 10 years before all the pieces come together: a stable, healthy environment; a secure, healthy family system and couple relationship; and a strong, healthy, autonomous sense of self.

ASSESSMENT: HOW TO LISTEN TO AND THINK ABOUT FAMILIES IN RECOVERY

As we said earlier, we started this project with strong biases and we ended this project with strong biases. As interpreters of data, particularly qualitative data—the family stories—we brought our individual theories and experiences, both personal and professional. We spent 5 years watching and listening to every tape, every family, transcribing their responses to our semistructured interview word for word. We listened with multiple theories in mind, charting theme, content, structure, and process across the three domains. We started with the developmental model for the individual and ended up with a more complex, multileveled theory, still grounded in stages and process.

There might well be other interpretations than ours; there certainly could be other interpretations with a different organizing lens than loss of control, abstinence, and a developmental perspective. These core principles, in addition to the other assumptions we listed in Chapter 1, shape assessment and intervention. Otherwise, the therapist may be working against the natural flow of recovery. The developmental theory emerges from the stories of families who have lived with alcoholism and identify themselves as recovering.

We have already said—and repeated—how important we think it is for therapists to know what a normal process of recovery is. That includes how difficult it is and how long it takes. The primary focus of this book is to outline and literally "map out" what recovery is, what happens and what is normal during the course of recovery. The task of the therapist follows from the stage and task of the recovery process for the particular patient(s) and the particular family.

While we are not offering a "how to" manual for therapists, we do believe in the value of therapeutic help all along the way. It simply must follow from the needs of the individuals and the family, which are often complex and even contradictory. In the short run, what is best for one person may not seem best for everyone else or the family as a whole, which poses a challenge for the therapist. Sometimes the best clinical intervention is to serve as a "holder" and a teacher, helping the family weather massive disruption and radical change while reassuring family members that what they are experiencing is normal. It is neither possible nor wise, at some points, to try to help them "build" anything, because tearing down and "collapse" of unsound structures are what is needed. But how do we help them do this and prevent further damage to their children? By education, support, and active intervention to ensure that children are not neglected or abandoned. Families generally don't make it through this crisis without lots of help, which we encourage and facilitate.

How does the therapist think about assessment and intervention, both short term and long term, within this perspective? In a broad sense, the assessment process is ongoing, from the first contact to termination. The therapist monitors the normal process of growth and watches for gaps or ruptures in development that may require intervention or repair. This includes a regular check on the daily recovery program for all family members; an assessment of the family's adjustments to abstinence, with attention to major problems; and a family history, past and present, including trauma, that may interfere with progress. Therapist monitoring may be focused and direct, taking a drinking or recovery history, for example, or, more global and in the background, as the therapist hears data about drinking that fills in a portrait of addiction over time. Intervention (i.e., the therapist's response), direct or indirect, follows from assessment.

In a global sense, the therapist is always considering what is positive, healthy, and belongs to a forward-moving developmental process, on the one hand and what is problematic, an obstacle, or resistance to movement toward or in recovery, on the other. What defenses are used by individuals or family in the service of maintaining movement in recovery and what defenses work against this positive flow? As we have said, this determination is often counterintuitive. For example, family members may complain that the alcoholic is no fun anymore, that this abstinent state fills their lives with tension, a problem they want fixed. The therapist may ask how it was before and what's missing besides fun, and empathize with how hard it is to live with the tension. The therapist may add what a hard time new recovery is when no one knows what's happening or what to do. The therapist may also wonder if family members are afraid the alcoholic will drink again. Sometimes the complaints mask the fear that none of this will last ("so we might as well get it [the uncertainty or tension] over with"). The therapist can make this interpretation and talk with the family about how they can live with this new uncertainty. The therapist does not join the family in viewing the tension as a problem to be fixed.

In some cases, a similar complaint indicates a different issue. For example, the family may resist recovery because it awakens feelings of loss and anger. If the therapist recognizes this and points it out to the family, they can begin to better understand how to bear their loss. In the next section, we'll meet a family whose members typify this kind of resistance.

The therapist must always remember that the drinking family system produces an unhealthy situation, although no one in the family may see it that way. Ironically, the newly recovering family is just as likely to fit mental health criteria for pathology as the drinking family. The therapist listens for information within the three domains that confirms the family's adaptations to drinking and to becoming an alcoholic family. For example, the therapist hears that there is a lot of parental arguing and constant tension that contribute to a chronically traumatic environment. The therapist then hears evidence of a tightening, restrictive system that reflects a growing defensiveness. The kids say that they can't bring friends home or that they're told not to talk about the family. Finally, the therapist hears that individuals are showing significant signs of stress—an increase in illness, or absences from school and work. Individuals are depressed and anxious, and they can't say why. This is a family that has "turned toward alcohol" (Brown, 1985). Now, normal thinking, affect, and behavior reinforce the maintenance of pathology.

These adaptations may have included the ability to function, and even to function reasonably well for some time, while bypassing or denying problems with drinking and the consequences of drinking. At this point, people often have no conscious awareness of what is being denied, repressed, and explained away. The therapist uses these data to anticipate resistance to recovery, particularly what some AA members call "romanticizing the past." Families suffering with abstinence may long for the old state of drinking and denial. Facing reality is just too hard. The therapist helps them recall what drinking was really like and how and why they got to recovery.

Since new recovery can feel and look worse for most families, the therapist must be able to assess the underlying current; the therapist needs to identify signs of attachment to recovery with simultaneous detachment from the pathology of drinking. The therapist charts the initial adjustment to abstinence and the steps the family makes to secure an abstinent foundation, all of which may seem more disturbed and problematic than the drinking. The therapist must tolerate the anxiety of the family and their pressure to fix it all so they can return to what they see as their normal state.

By holding this global view, or faith in the recovery process, the therapist can better function in the many roles required. He or she may need to challenge, cajole, coach, support, or interpret; or focus on one family member while letting another hold still for a while. Understanding the anxiety and tension that accompanies this initial recovery stage (for some, this period extends for quite a while) will help the therapist allow the family to weather uncertainty.

Based on the therapist's understanding of the progress and/or resistance within domains and stages, the therapist can use these data to determine the clinical "next step." When and how should the therapist intervene? Should he or she use a behavioral, cognitive, dynamic or systems focus of interpretation or active intervention? Clearly, all these decisions need to be based on the therapist's assessment of the particular family. For example, how does the therapist know when a challenge or direct intervention is called for or when a more watchful, extended view, or an interpretive frame is the better next step? In working with a drinking family, the "next step" may be an acute intervention, such as immediate hospitalization, or a decision to wait for more devastation to occur and the family's defenses to weaken. Working with a family in the early weeks of abstinence may require direct advice, support, and reinforcement for abstinent behaviors, a coaching role. Much later the therapist assumes a more reflective, interpretive role. These next steps are viewed within the context of domain and stage in the long-term frame. There are so many ups and downs and so much trauma in recovery that it is too easy to jump to the wrong conclusions unless the therapist maintains a vision of both the short-term and the long-term process.

THE ORGANIZING FOCUS
OF ALCOHOL ADDICTION: GUIDELINES

When the therapist takes a history, or listens session to session with addiction or recovery as an organizing principle (Brown, 1985, 1995a, 1995b; Steinglass et al., 1987; Steinglass, 1980; Amodeo, 1995a; 1995b; Zweben, 1995), different data and a different perspective emerge. It is no wonder so many therapists have said, and still say, that they never heard anything about drinking in their work with patients. Perhaps the patient refuses to talk about his or her drinking, but therapists also misinterpret data that could give them solid information about addiction because they are listening to and thinking about the patient within a different organizing schema.

It may be that a couple talks only about the chaos and fighting in their family and the therapist never asks about alcohol use. The intervention then may focus on helping the couple learn better communication skills. Or the therapist may find out about alcohol use but decides that the drinking is a response to marital problems. The couple believe the same thing. If the therapist were to see alcohol in its organizing role in the couple relationship, he or she would have avoided reinforcing the family's defenses and perhaps his or her own as well. Marital problems might have led to drinking in the beginning, but over time drinking has reinforced old problems and caused new ones (Vaillant, 1983; Levin, 1987, 1998; Van Bree, 1995).

In listening with an "alcohol focus," the therapist gathers data, directly and indirectly, regarding the family members' relationship to drinking and recovery. Is this a drinking family? Does anyone identify drinking as a problem? Is this a recovering family? If so, who identifies as "being in recovery," who doesn't, why, and how, are all important assessment questions. Is alcoholism, or family alcoholism, organizing a recovery process? There is great variability between families, depending on multiple factors. For example, is one or both parents alcoholic? Do one or both parents enter recovery—at the same time or at different times? What are the ages of children during the drinking and entry into recovery? Was the entry into recovery acute, with crisis and systems collapse, or was it a long, extended process, one person after another? Is recovery a one-person story with the rest of the family not involved? Whatever the pattern, is there support, warmth and an environment and system that encourage personal autonomy and growth? Or is there conflict, anger, and unresolved tension?

The therapist wonders what it means to individuals and the family as a whole to think of themselves as "alcoholic" or as an "alcoholic family in recovery." Is there resistance to identifying alcoholism or moving toward recovery? Is there resistance to being in recovery? Does resistance facilitate or inhibit growth?

Understanding the meaning of alcoholism is vital as it helps the therapist assess and challenge denial. When a family is still drinking, the idea of being alcoholic, or an alcoholic family, is going to be bad. Patients routinely say that being an alcoholic means they are weak, a failure, or "just like my parents." In the context of evaluation and ongoing therapy, exploring these meanings will help the therapist and patient(s) understand the dynamics and defenses of drinking. No one, consciously, wants to be an alcoholic. Nor does anyone, consciously, want to be a partner to an alcoholic. Rarely does anyone decide to be an alcoholic, as if he or she were choosing a career. Many people say they believed, in retrospect, that becoming alcoholic was nonetheless inevitable.

Therapists assume that the reality of alcoholism will not be welcome news. Thus, as they develop the portrait of addiction and the nature of defense, they are also anticipating the kinds of difficulties, including resistance, that the family will have in recovery, based on this information: how the drinking worked; what it meant; what defenses and beliefs organized the family to maintain the drinking; what the environment was like; how the system adapted itself to maintain drinking; and what being in recovery means.

In addition, the therapist takes a historical view. What has been the role and meaning of alcohol to this family and the parents' families of origin? Is alcoholism a tradition, carried on for generations, or something new to this family? Is there a history of past trauma, or other psychiatric conditions, such as depression and anxiety disorders? What role has alcohol played in coping with other problems?

In the next section, we'll hear the stories of four families in recovery to illustrate the process of family recovery from an alcohol focus.

THE NEED FOR THERAPIST FLEXIBILITY

Earlier, we emphasized the importance of flexibility in the therapist role. The therapist works as a monitor, charting normal movement in recovery and spotting problems that require clinical intervention, including a recommendation for intensive therapy. The therapist also functions as a coach and supporter, helping people cope with the radical changes and disruption by mapping out the terrain and providing concrete education. The therapist is a resource person, wearing any number of hats, sometimes all at the same time and all in one session.

This variability in role also applies to the theoretical frame. As we've already noted, most therapists in mental health disciplines (psychiatry, psychology, social work, and marriage and family counselors) are trained in one primary theory of development and change that informs their clinical work—how they listen and what interventions they make—to a significant degree. They may identify themselves as behaviorists, cognitive psychologists, cognitive-behaviorists, or psychodynamically oriented or systems specialists. Rarely do therapists identify with all of these schools and use the principles from each in an integrated way in their work with patients. In fact, there is much competition and animosity between schools about the validity and usefulness of their theories and methods.

Addiction counselors are also trained in a limited way. Their specialized training and treatment perspective often has its roots in

AA experience. Many of these therapists are recovering alcoholics, coalcoholics, or adult children of alcoholics whose professional theory and practice have been greatly influenced by their personal experiences. Although they usually hold a long-term view of recovery from their knowledge of AA, they do not have clinical experience working with recovering people over the long term. Like mental health, the professional addiction treatment models have focused only on the acute, relatively short-term transition from drinking to abstinence.

The emphasis on narrow, specialized training can be a major problem for all therapists, from all disciplines, if they do not have a working knowledge of all schools, an appreciation for the validity of the varying theories and methods, and knowledge of integrating these approaches in working with the alcoholic family.

The therapist needs to be flexible in practice, able to intervene at concrete behavioral levels one moment while shifting to a reflective, analytic stance in the next. Preferably, the therapist should also be comfortable holding multiple roles: to give support, direct instruction, and advice; to maintain a more traditional neutral stance, not taking a position or giving advice; to act as a supportive coach, cheering the hard work onward; to challenge and to wonder about thinking, motivation, resistance, and defense; and to interpret individual and systems dynamics.

In a narrow framework, this kind of flexibility and multiple focus might be viewed by some schools as therapist resistance or countertransference. However, in working with addiction and recovery, the therapist may positively function in all these modes in a single session, thereby helping the family stabilize in recovery and contributing to cohesiveness in treatment rather than fragmentation. It is supportive of both the here-and-now focus and the longer-term underlying process of recovery.

The therapist, like the patient, holds the acceptance of loss of control and abstinence as the primary organizers of listening and intervention. Following the developmental view, the therapist initially supports active behavior change as the patient and family shift from an all-absorbing focus on the drinking system to individual attention to learning abstinent behaviors. Families are also focused on cognitive change, challenging denial about the past and building new identities in the present as alcoholics or coalcoholics. An in-depth psychodynamic view may be necessary if resistance to abstinence or recovery and the new learning is strong, or if issues from the past interfere with people's ability to remain abstinent or to develop a commitment and attachment to recovery. Being the adult child of an alcoholic (ACOA) is one example. Growing up with parental alcoholism will have a profound impact on such individuals' view about their own alcoholism and recovery, both as individuals and as a family. Therapists may also focus on the system, explaining to the family why everything feels so disrupted, or not, and what is normal in this radical process of change. The therapist provides information all along the way to help ease the buildup of intolerable anxiety about all this change and the family systems vacuum created by the end of drinking.

In Early Recovery and Ongoing Recovery, with abstinence stable, the behavioral and cognitive emphasis assumes a more stable role as well, making room for psychodynamic exploration. Individuals, through working the 12 steps and perhaps psychotherapy, undertake a rigorous, ongoing process of self-examination. During this time, they may also begin to explore their couple relationship, past and present. The primary attention to the individual now expands to include the system.

In Part III, where we focus on more detailed assessment, we will describe the domains, stages, and primary tasks, and present a summary of the treatment focus at each stage

USING THE FAMILY INTERVIEW IN THE CLINICAL SETTING

The family research interview (see Appendix A) is a powerful intervention and therapeutic tool. Indeed, our research families were both excited and anxious about participating in the study. The interview provided the first opportunity to tell their story and yet also open up still-undiscovered feelings and memories.

Many of our couples and families told us that they had not purposely held back information from each other; they didn't have a format, and they didn't have the idea of a "story" of couple and family recovery. Our questions offered many respondents their first opportunity to think about themselves as a "couple, or family, in recovery," and to say aloud, within the safety and structure of a research interview, what it was like for each of them. Many had not talked together because they had done such a good job of "separating," learning in the beginning months and years of recovery to focus on themselves. Though some grew closer as a couple through sharing what they were learning in their individual programs, they did not learn the skills or feel the safety to open up certain difficult issues between them. For example, with time, most of our couples illustrated a tremendous shift in decision making about practical family matters, shifting from a one-person, dictatorial system, to a shared, equal partnership. But this dramatic equalization in power did not necessarily transfer to emotional issues, particularly those involving sex and anger. For many couples, these issues remained untouched and unresolved long into recovery. Here, the therapist can help, utilizing traditional psychodynamic therapy as well as more practical couples therapy interventions.

Another surprise was the interview itself. After we had completed interviews of several research families we knew that the interview was a powerful "intervention." Similar to a detailed clinical family history but focused on drinking and recovery, the interview gave people a new perspective on how to think about themselves. All but one family (51 out of 52) said it had been very helpful to them. (Several years later, this family said that they too were glad they had participated. It had opened up a well of pain, but over time they found it useful.) Sometimes the couple said they learned a lot about themselves and each other, and occasionally they said they learned nothing new. But the opportunity to talk and to share their experience was important and valuable to them. One family brought intense unresolved conflicts into the interview, laid them out, and left as angry as they had been for years of recovery. If they had not already been in therapy, which ironically had stirred up the deep, underlying pain, we would have recommended it.

It was clear to us that the interview was a very useful clinical tool. It helped the families construct a narrative, or "family story," putting names to memories and feelings. In this way, it solidified the realities of both drinking and recovery that many had already constructed in an individual AA or Al-Anon story. Several families said the process gave them a bridge to begin talking with each other about their lives as a couple. A number said they had approached problems between them by each "going to a meeting." Early on, that was immensely helpful, but later, with years of abstinence, many of our families needed the help of the interview structure and of third parties (sometimes of us, as researchers and, in other settings, as clinicians) to work things out together. Some had found tremendous individual growth through their 12-step programs and/or therapy and/or religion, but they did not know how to come back together as a couple or were too afraid to try.

Our interview served an important function of helping the family structure its own history around alcohol and alcoholism as a central organizing principle. When people said things for the first time, it made them real. Sometimes long-held secrets were revealed. In many cases, telling their story of family alcoholism and recovery facilitated new dialogue.

One 20-year-old son said he had been angry with his father for 15 years. He then described being 5 years old, thrown across the room, into the wall, by his drunken father. Dad, Mom, and two other grown children sat still. Father said he did not remember this violence, but he believed his son. He looked directly at him and apologized.

These children proceeded to describe to us how close they had become since their father stopped drinking almost 3 years earlier. Though all the children are grown, with families of their own, they now come to their parents' home nearly every weekend, literally to be with the father they never had.

We suggest that the family interview be a routine part of "recovery monitoring" following abstinence. It can be seen as a periodic "health and well-being" check to help the family chart movement, identify problems, and anticipate hurdles, both those that are normal and expected and those that are particular to this family. For example, adults who grew up with alcoholic parents will have to cope with and explore their own past and present as ACOAs. Sometimes they must do this in order to be abstinent, and sometimes they can only maintain abstinence by postponing the work of childhood trauma (Brown, 1994). The therapist monitors the developmental process within each domain and across stages, watching closely for current difficulties and determining when issues from the past need attention.

A MAP

When we began this project we decided to write a curriculum for families in recovery based on our idea that knowing what is normal in recovery and knowing what to expect would be helpful to families. As we noted earlier, we called the curriculum MAPS, short for "Maintaining Abstinence Programs." The acronym fit our views about process well: we would "map out" the terrain of recovery.

In this book we will literally map out a process of family recovery: What is it? How do we define it? How do couples and families define it? What are the similarities between families, and therefore common issues and themes that emerge, and what are the differences? Are there commonalities that we will also call "normal"?

These are stories—family stories of living with alcoholism. There is a rhythm and an order: What happened? What was it like? How did it feel? Who was there? Who wasn't there? One of our families, in recovery for many years, described the impact of looking back through the family photo album:

> "We paused at the portrait of a wedding party and were stunned by who was missing: Uncle Ray died in a drunk-driving accident, cousin Sophie was far away, strung out on drugs. Grandma had just died. At the time, we thought it was a stroke. Really, she had fallen down the stairs, drunk, and died from head injury. Staring at that picture, the damage, and the losses from generations of alcoholism stood out. It was pretty shocking. Then we looked around at each other—who was here today and who was sober? We've come a long way."

What we learned in our research and in testing our curriculum with families became the developmental model of family recovery. We hope it will be reassuring, supportive, and helpful to families, who, just like therapists, may misinterpret the short-term results, deciding that recovery has failed, because they have no map and no experience of a bigger picture that shows how things often get worse before they get better.

What have we emphasized so far? Complexity, disruption, ongoing trauma, necessary changes that can inadvertently cause additional trauma; systems collapse; the danger of child neglect and abandonment in recovery. Where is the hope in all of this? Hope underlies every family story. You will hear it as families tell what happened to them and how they see it and feel about it today.

We are describing a difficult process of change that is not the "outcome" people expect, not the solution to the "problem" that everyone wanted, and not "happy-ever-after." So let us say now and repeat it throughout the book: abstinence is a good thing, a wonderful, positive event, though getting there is almost always devastating. Recovery too is a wonderful, positive process, though it is also difficult, painful, and traumatic. As our research families in recovery told us what it was like during the drinking, what happened to them, and what it has been like in recovery, they expressed a continuing wonder and awe about the gifts they have been given. So, when we talk about problems, about how hard a road it is, remember that the overriding experience has been very positive. Our families in recovery are deeply grateful. They would not give this up, and they would not change it. But it has been hard.

Let us move to Part II, in which we present the shortened summaries of four families in recovery who illustrate different stages, issues, and tasks in recovery. We quote liberally from the interviews to let the theory come alive through the voices and interactions of the families. We want the reader to get the "feel" for the family together, talking with each other.

It is important to remember that we were researchers, with these families for one 3-hour interview. Otherwise, the reader may think us callous and heartless, as we sometimes did. It was often hard to stick with the structured interview when we empathized with people who were feeling deeply. In many cases, people wanted help. They volunteered because they knew, often unconsciously, that they needed to open up, and they did. At the end of the interview, having completed our task as researchers, we talked with the families. Sometimes we donned our clinical hats and gave feedback and suggestions for additional help, which always included AA and Al-Anon if people were not involved, and strong support for continuing in these 12-step programs if they were already members. We also recommended psychotherapy.

Next, in Part III, we provide a framework for assessment: an overview of the domains and stages that compose the developmental model of recovery, reflecting back to these families as examples. Finally, we look at a variety of factors that influence recovery.

In Part IV, we shift from theory back to the voices of the families, who tell us their stories and illustrate the stages and process in detail.

PART TWO

Stories of Families in Recovery

CHAPTER THREE

Transition and Early Recovery

THE CORWINS AND THE TURNERS

In this chapter and the next, we'll meet four families with different lengths of abstinence and different patterns and experiences of alcoholism and recovery. They demonstrate the successes and problems, ups and downs, in the natural, normal flow of recovery. These families will show us through the tasks, focus, and common themes that arise during this phase.

The details of these families are real, but we have changed identifying information in order to maintain the confidentiality of our volunteers. We will summarize their stories by loosely following the interview questions, which are found in Appendix A. We will also comment about how we listen, the meaning we derive, and how we would use what we learned clinically.

THE CORWINS: 5 MONTHS' ABSTINENCE— TRANSITION STAGE

The Corwins, Josh (55) and Lisa (52), live in a small town in Central Oregon. Their daughter, Cary (28), saw a flier about our research at church and urged her parents to participate. The couple agreed if Cary and her brother, Ken (26), would come too. Josh and Lisa have been married for 31 years. At the time of the interview, Josh had been abstinent for 5 months.

When the researcher asked the first question, "What was it like for each of you during the drinking, and what was it like for your family as a whole?," Cary jumped in to answer. From the beginning of the interview, it was clear that she was desperately worried about her father and saw the interview as a way of saying so, hoping that he would seek additional help. Dad was only angrily and grudgingly attending AA, seeing Cary as the one who needed help. As you'll see, everyone needed help and no one was getting any.

CARY: It wasn't a family. There was no cohesion, no trust, no stability. Well, there was stability actually—I always knew my father would be drinking. They would be arguing, and my dad would be hassling me. I knew what to expect and it wasn't good.

KEN: I was bothered by his drinking. I can remember back to 6 years old—I was upset. I knew it wasn't normal, and I wanted it to be different.

It was normal too. I had friends over, I went to school and I went to other alcoholic households that were more severe. Ours had periodic disruption. I can remember more as a teen—I felt distinctly uncomfortable with Dad's drinking.

CARY: He would joke; we all did. And then he would change and become aggressive; he picked on us; we all felt on edge. If things were calm, you wanted to keep them that way.

I used to cook for him, though I'd say I didn't want to. He'd say I was lazy and how come I didn't want to do things for him? He used to watch all the glasses carefully and be upset if others got more.

Cary and Ken show us that they can label their dad's drinking, remember what it was like, talk about it with us, though not with each other, and have feelings about it. But the talking and remembering are very new. It is only in the last 5 months, since their dad participated in a treatment program, that Cary and Ken can speak openly.

Lisa is becoming aware of her denial as she recalls how she thought about things, and she is beginning to question why she stayed with Josh. The erosion of denial is an incremental process. It begins during drinking and moves people to abstinence. But it is not over.

The challenge of denial and all distorted thinking continue long into recovery.

With 5 months' abstinence for Josh, Lisa's dawning awareness is a window, a small opening that casts a new light but does not yet alter Lisa's view of herself or others. Lisa shows us how captive she was to not seeing alcoholism. For many, denial is like a fog that thickens the atmosphere and narrows vision. Denial often lifts like fog as well, slowly dissipating as individuals become ready to "see" more clearly.

LISA: (*to Cary*) You told the shrink you were concerned about your dad's drinking in the fourth grade. You were more honest than you remember. For a long time, I thought we all drank too much until Josh stood out. I don't come from an alcoholic family, so I didn't recognize alcoholism and I wasn't looking for it. Josh told me when we met that he didn't want to become an alcoholic, and I didn't get it. The first time he told me he hadn't had a drink in 2 days I was surprised.

I thought we had a normal suburban life. We drank, but so did everyone. We went to work and had a good life—lots of friends, lots of partying, and it all seemed normal to me. Then it crept up on me that something was wrong. We fought all the time, and I started to want to get away. I was upset with myself because I couldn't figure out why I was still around. I'm still asking myself: Why didn't I walk away?

Then she gives us a clue: she distanced herself from Josh, investing in her work and her own life instead of him.

LISA: I decided to get involved with my work and lead my own life. I remember saying to myself that I couldn't leave because I loved my house.

Lisa's "it crept up on me . . . " illustrates a softening in her defenses and beginning changes in her thinking. She was preparing to acknowledge the reality of Josh's drinking as she was becoming able to depend less on him, changes that were evolving unconsciously.

LISA: There were signs, but I didn't pay attention. I was kidding myself. It was on and off and not major. When I finally knew there was a problem, I decided I'd live with it and just do what I do. Finally I couldn't take it anymore.

Cary coped by believing that her mother was the cause of her father's drinking. In this way, she focused her emotional hurt and anguish about both of her parents onto her mother and, idealizing her father, vested her hopes and dependency in him. To maintain such a positive view of her father, she had to minimize the realities and damaging effects of his drinking.

CARY: I had a better childhood than lots of my friends. I had a good relationship with my dad: he was always there, and our only problem was the drinking. It bothered me when I thought about it, so I tried not to.

Cary illustrates some of the defenses necessary for the child of an alcoholic. Through minimization, she softens the harshness of reality. In addition, she screens out thoughts and feelings about a reality she cannot speak of or change. In such a captive relationship and environment, in which reality must be denied and lived with at the same time, she must alter her perceptions, explanations, and affective receptivity to incoming data in order to maintain attachment (Brown, 1988, 1991b, 1991c). The child's defensive accommodations become a "false self," or "defensive self," an overlay constructed by children to cope with the trauma and the pathogenic, pathological basis of attachment (Brown, 1991b, 1991c, 1995c).

Cary reinforces her need to believe in her Dad and to hold a positive view of him.

CARY: My mom got depressed. It was scary for me. We went from a pretty good relationship and a solid safe place which I counted on to nothing. We fought and my mom said it was all my fault. I went to live with friends for a while. (*to her dad*) You were drunk most days but usually not sloppy. Then there were the bad ones. One time I came home from school, and we all got ripped together. We just drank—to be attached.

Although Cary is defensive about her father and minimizes the impact of his drinking, she also shows us that she knows and remembers a lot that she can speak about when given permission, such as in this family interview.

In addition, Cary illustrates a central truth about alcohol and some families: Adults and children frequently end up drinking together because any semblance of close relationship evolves around alcohol. Children often can't wait to join the grown-ups; drinking lets everyone maintain denial while it dulls the painful reality of being a sober child, alone with drunken, out-of-control parents.

Josh is quiet, listening to the others remember what happened. They describe several years of descent into chronic, severe alcoholism. The family was now organized and dominated by Josh's drinking. The interviewer asked, "What led to the end?" and Josh described his long road toward "hitting bottom." As things got worse, he maintained his belief that his problem was not alcohol. By now, his family knew otherwise.

Why did it take so long for the Corwins to "get it," to see that it was alcohol? It took so long because no one wanted to know. Lisa is just now asking herself why she stayed, why she went along with it. One of the reasons it takes so long to get to the "bottom" is because families are doing all they can to stay together, all they can to make things OK. That often means not rocking the boat and not insisting on labeling reality—the reality of drinking—if others maintain it isn't so. People want happy families, and they will go to great lengths to believe that's exactly what they have.

JOSH: I was hospitalized several times for detox. Then I was put on the psych ward for manic–depression and depression. This covered several years—we all thought I wasn't really an alcoholic; it was something else which the doctors kept trying to figure out.

Josh illustrates a significant professional dilemma: the need to sort out which came first, alcoholism or something else, in order to assign primary, secondary, or tertiary diagnostic rank. The ranking usually dictates the focus of treatment, which creates a danger of reinforcing the denial system of the alcoholic. There is some other problem that is causing the individual to drink; or the individual drinks to cope with, or solve, the "primary" problem. The therapist takes the view that solving the "other" problem will also solve the need to drink. Other psychiatric problems may predate alcoholism, other problems may mask alcoholism, and other problems result from alcoholism. The difficulty of sorting out cause and effect is the "catch-22" of what is called "dual diagnosis" (Nace, 1995). Regardless of any other condition or diagnosis, alcoholism must be seen as "primary," or as a separate, "coexisting" disorder. If not, it will likely not be treated directly; the professional is then caught in exactly the same "thinking disorder" and denial as the alcoholic and family, looking for "something else" to treat with the expectation that the drinking "problem" will then be solved.

LISA: Then you got your first DUI [driving under the influence charge], another detox, another DUI. You went to AA for a while, which was good, but nothing changed. What a difference it is now. I went to see the first doctor and called in the family. We told Josh he had to go to treatment for alcoholism or I would leave.

JOSH: I was aware for a long time that I drank a lot and could drink a lot. I was depressed, and I wasn't sure if it related to drinking. I took a bunch of medications and stopped them all. I'm confused about how much alcohol was involved with the depression. I drank to get numb and to feel better. It was out of control.

Some people turn to alcohol to treat depression or other emotional problems. Alcohol may cover these psychological difficulties at first, providing positive reinforcement for the individual to keep drinking as a solution to other problems. But alcohol is also a depressant, which will eventually intensify the problems it was supposed to fix and cause new depression and other problems related to the consequences of drinking. It is a vicious cycle that becomes impossible to sort out.

INTERVIEWER: Were you ever worried?

JOSH: Yes; when you know it's out of control. When you know you have to drink more to quiet the shakes or you have to go get medication. It's not easy to see. The easiest thing is to keep on drinking—see where it's going.

When Josh tells us that "the drinking was out of control" we know the drinking had a life of its own. Josh has alcoholism.

JOSH: I can't be clear when I was in serious trouble. Years ago six or seven drinks a day was normal. I didn't perceive it as heavy drinking, but now I do.

From the vantage point of abstinence, Josh can revise his definition of what constitutes "too much" alcohol. In his view, "normal" could not also be "too much," so he could not see six or seven drinks as a problem.

The interviewer was struck by the continuing isolation and anger of everyone in this family, including Josh. So, even though she already knew he attended AA, she asked, "What about AA and Al-Anon?" We see that Lisa is resistant to being engaged in recovery for herself. So is Josh.

LISA: I have a friend who's pushing me to go, but I haven't found a group I feel comfortable in. I went a long time ago and didn't like it. I reached out for help in a crisis. The counselor told me to go to Al-Anon, and I was angry.

JOSH: We came to this project for Cary. She wants to be involved with ACOA [meetings].

We see Josh shift the focus to his daughter, another sign of his resistance to being engaged in recovery for himself.

INTERVIEWER: (to Cary) What did you see about this project that would be helpful?

CARY: When Dad was in treatment a counselor told me it would be important for the family to continue recovery afterward in order to help my dad. I also thought we could help others. I want to do whatever I can to help my dad not drink.

I went to ACOA meetings and was terrified. I felt sorry for these people whose experience seemed so much more extreme than mine. I don't feel screwed up by it, though I should have gotten some help when Dad was drinking.

Again we see Cary minimizing her own feelings and experiences as she maintains her focus on her father. We understand why she is worried. He is not invested in his recovery, and Cary knows it. In a clinical setting, the therapist might explore the relationship between Cary's attachment to her father and her need to continue to feel responsible for him.

JOSH: I was upset a lot in all my treatments. I don't like authority, and I hate bureaucracy. I was angry that they told me what to do.

We see Josh's resistance to following guidelines or suggestions. He maintains his anger at authorities whom he perceives have more control, which keeps Josh from investing in himself and his own growth. In a clinical setting, we might inquire how he feels about accepting loss of control and about being an alcoholic.

The interviewer then asks what life is like now.

LISA: We spend more time together; before, Josh was in front of the TV.

JOSH: It's qualitatively better. I'm more available, more in touch.

But then Josh and Lisa add, almost in unison, "We're not open; we don't share, and we never did."

JOSH: The way it is is survivable. There's a reasonable comfort level. I'd like to see it improve. The absence of drinking makes the absence between us clearer.

LISA: It's survivable; I'm not open.

This is the first mention of problems between Josh and Lisa now, though we can feel and hear the anger and tension. The interviewer asks questions about changes in family function and about the significance of recovery in their lives. We learn that the Corwins are not in a recovery process: Josh is "dry," and no one is moving or changing. The family is in a holding zone, dominated by anger. We know Josh and the family are in danger of relapse, as there has been very little change and angry feelings are building.

In a clinical setting, we would share all these observations and offer suggestions to the family if they were receptive.

INTERVIEWER: How has decision making changed?

JOSH: It hasn't changed; there is no difference.

We know that it takes a long time in recovery for decision processes, which reflect systemic structure, to change. Here we see that the family system is operating in old patterns that have not collapsed nor changed. This is a system dominated by a brooding, long-standing hostility and anger.

INTERVIEWER: How much is recovery a part of your lives?

JOSH: I'm more involved; go to meetings. Others are coming along for the ride. Recovery is because of me.

LISA: It's not a huge part. We never talk about it. The family is better because you're recovering, Josh.

We see that Lisa is angry and self-protective. She cannot become engaged in her own recovery process. This is part of why Transition is so hard. Both Josh and Lisa recognize and feel the vacuum between them, which they have no way of resolving *as a couple* without returning to drinking and the denial system they shared for many years. Neither can go back at this point, but they cannot change either unless and until they can shift the focus off the other and onto themselves as individuals.

Cary shares her view of her father now:

CARY: I talk about it, but he won't talk. It's easier to ask for money. I'm interested, I want to know, but he won't talk. My relationship is better with Dad. I like being with him, and he contributes to the conversation—more than joking or correcting what I said. He's happier, more alive. But I'm not familiar with this person; this is different, brand new. I don't feel secure. I get anxious. I found a bottle of wine in the refrigerator, and it sent terror through me. I'm very watchful. I remember the sights and the sounds, and I'm concerned when I'm not with him.

Cary illustrates the chronic anxiety the ACOA often feels—anxiety about the past, about change now, and about what this new person, her father, is like and will be like. She cannot focus on herself, independent of worrying about him. From an alcohol-focused perspective, we share Cary's concern: what is a bottle of wine doing in the refrigerator? Cary seems to be the only person paying attention to alcohol, a responsibility that is, of course, not hers. Although we would recommend that she focus on herself, attending 12-step programs and psychotherapy, we can also see why she can't. She needs reassurance that someone else will look after her father before she can let go of her vigilance of him. We also surmise that her sense of responsibility is closely linked to her attachment to him, which operates unconsciously (as well as consciously) and thus will not be easily challenged.

INTERVIEWER: Do you see that there have been stages in your recovery?

LISA: In the first part of sobriety I used to get nervous when you'd come home, but not now. I used to have to call Josh in the mornings, but now I can call him at night and I like it. It was wonderful when Josh was in the hospital. It was time to step back and feel wonderful. I wasn't sure I wanted him to come back. I didn't want the chaos. I told myself everything would be OK, and then after a month when it wasn't, I decided not to call.

Lisa illustrates the shock of abstinence for her and the shattering of illusions that followed. The beginning of abstinence is often very difficult because the reality is so different from people's expectations. The introduction to recovery—becoming abstinent—is often full of disappointment for all. This is particularly true if no one is invested in recovery. Abstinence is then likely to be a "white-knuckle" holding operation.

CARY: It was eggshells in the beginning; not wanting to mention alcohol.

And now we hear Josh's anger again:

JOSH: I don't see stages. I hate having people around the house. I'm self-centered.

We also hear Josh's edginess, his raw nerves. This is what has been called in AA a "dry drunk." Josh is experiencing the emotions and physical sensations that go along with drinking, but now minus alcohol. Sometimes people respond to this intense, uncomfortable state with a return to drinking.

INTERVIEWER: Do you have a family story of recovery?

JOSH: No. We don't like all the focus. I don't need people to ask me questions; I'm not into birthdays [sobriety anniversaries], and a lot of people don't even know. I don't look to other people for help. I know I should get a sponsor, but if you tell me to, I won't.

We continue to see Josh's anger and resistance. He does not want to talk with his family or us. We have a sense that abstinence feels like punishment and deprivation to him.

LISA: I judge how I feel according to him. I want to know how he's doing, but it's none of my business.

We also continue to see Lisa's inability to acknowledge herself. She remains focused on Josh, determining her own feelings through him.

At the end of the interview, Lisa, Cary, and Ken agree that they liked it. Cary says that it was the only way her father would talk. We feel serious concern. The Corwin family is holding onto a precarious abstinence and barely "surviving." We do not hear signs of a beginning building process of recovery, so we know the family has a rocky start. Josh is dry, but he is not in recovery; nor is anyone else.

In a recovery check, the therapist takes the family through each domain—the environment, the system, and the individuals—to assess movement and sees that there is no change process underway. The environment is dry, not wet, but still tense and permeated by hostility. The system and the individuals have not changed at all.

The therapist notes the strong signs of trouble: Josh is the only person in any recovery activities, and he is resisting; the others are all focused on him, with anger, worry, or both; the family is dominated by defense—everyone carries an air of impending doom as they sense the danger of relapse.

Therapists share their perceptions, outlining the absence of movement, the holes throughout each domain, and the danger of relapse. The therapist might also ask: What is in the way? What is holding family members back? Can the anger be faced, dealt with, or is it too entrenched, the glue of the couple bond? Another question, useful at any time, is to wonder what it would be like, for each person and the family as a whole, if movement was underway and holes were attended to? What would this kind of "success" look like and feel like? Many families are terrified of change and resist embracing recovery because of fear. Others are skeptical, still too close to the trauma of drinking, and cannot risk feeling hope or joining a recovery process.

THE TURNERS: 16 MONTHS' ABSTINENCE—
EARLY RECOVERY

The Turners, Hal (48) and Maggie (47), have been married for 20 years. They have three teenage children who are not part of the interview. Hal identifies himself as alcoholic with 1 year, 4 months' abstinence. Maggie and Hal attended a lecture at a Southern California treatment center and learned of the research. Hal was particularly interested in learning more about ACOAs, as his father and mother were alcoholics.

Following the same format for nearly all our families, the interviewer asks the first question: "What was it like for each of you during the drinking, and what was it like for you as a couple?" Hal and Maggie speak softly at first, with a dark, serious cast to their voices. Though they speak in hushed tones, they paint a picture full of intense emotion: sorrow, fear, anger, loss.

MAGGIE: Alcohol was always the center of our relationship. The first 3 years were positive, and then I began to see problems. Now I can see that alcohol was always there. He drank before lunch every day, and I became openly concerned. He couldn't run his business, shaking every morning. I got books about alcoholism. We both saw therapists, and he stopped drinking for a while. But there was so much tension, neither of us went to meetings, and we were isolated. I was no help. I needed Al-Anon.

At this point, Hal and Maggie were "dry" but not in a process of recovery. What they describe is the absence of alcohol.

HAL: We went to couples therapy, but it was no help. We were depressed, lifeless. I started drinking again.

MAGGIE: It was a sad, dark time. I was hyperalert for the sounds of drinking—the refrigerator door opening, ice. After I'd go to bed, he'd continue drinking. I always wondered if we'd be able to have conversations or if he'd be too drunk. I pulled away from him, as he was depressed. We became separate, parallel partners, isolated and self-sufficient. He became melancholy and drank more. I'd get up in the night to see if he was alive. One day I came home and there was a note he'd gone to the hospital. I felt incredible relief. But my hopes were dashed. He was a different person, withdrawn and not approachable.

Maggie describes how Hal was lost to alcohol when he was drinking and how he was lost to alcohol—to his focus on being in recovery—when he was newly abstinent. At the end of drinking and the beginning of abstinence (Transition) Hal was struggling within himself and was not available for an intimate partnership with Maggie. This is often very difficult to accept, for the couple and the therapist. The reality of separateness, both in the terrible downward slide to the "bottom" of drinking and the often terrible beginning days and weeks of abstinence, runs counter to everyone's belief about how things should be. In fact, neither partner is capable of a healthy, intimate bond at this point.

MAGGIE: When he was drunk he wasn't approachable either. Now, I resented his meetings every night. He had no time for me. First it was liquor, and now it was recovery. I didn't count. I still struggle with it. He has to remember he's alcoholic, and I sometimes forget. I went to Al-Anon a few times then, but I was too impatient. I wanted my husband, and I didn't want to wait.

Maggie, like Lisa, was angry. She wanted a relationship with Hal, which wasn't possible in the old way, before problems with alcohol, or in any way now.

HAL: I started therapy before I got sober and I continued in recovery. We went together to a family support group for 1 year.

MAGGIE: When the supports ended, I felt lost and became very depressed.

Hal then reflects about himself:

HAL: I was drinking alcoholically by my 20s. My parents drank and I simply followed along. Alcohol lifted my mood. I was very successful in my work, but the more successful I got, the more unhappy I became.

My world fell apart and I became a chronic drunk. I followed my parents again, though I swore I'd never be like them. I drank to oblivion every night.

We hear the profound impact of living with alcoholic parents. From this comment, we can surmise that Hal's development—his childhood experiences, his sense of self, and his identification with his parents—was probably shaped significantly by alcoholism. In a clinical setting, we would routinely listen for the organizing, developmental influence of alcohol and alcoholism and the need for intervention at this early dynamic level. To what degree would a focus on the past (i.e., growing up with parental alcoholism) help Hal and us understand his resistance to recovery?

HAL: The first time I went to several treatment programs, but I never followed treatment with AA. I thought AA was too much like church, which I didn't like at all.

Hal illustrates his continuing denial. He did not see that treatment is a time-limited event while recovery is ongoing.

HAL: I was barely functional in work. And I was miserable. I didn't know what I wanted to do. I always thought I had to do what my parents wanted.

Here we note a reference to his parents. Again, we feel the intensity of long-carried emotion and conflict.

HAL: Everything progressed. I was physically addicted to alcohol and very depressed. My daughter stopped speaking to me, and I went on a binge. I knew I was going to die, and I went to the hospital.

Hal defines his moment of "surrender": he was going to die and he made a move for help.

HAL: The first 2 months I was jubilant. Then I was numb. Then the anger came. I had a lot of feelings.

MAGGIE: He was angry with everyone, and he was verbally abusive to me.

HAL: I didn't grasp that there was anything wrong with who I was and the way I looked at the world. I had a crisis. I was feeling very anxious and raw. Who I'd been was no good, and I didn't know where I was going. One day I blew up. We had a bad fight and I walked out.

I think I might have opened too much in these first months. I was taking classes and attending workshops on ACOA. All these feelings were coming up for me, and I had no place to go with them.

The soft, hushed tone of voice we have been hearing so far now make sense. Hal and Maggie had just been through a terrible crisis. Hal broke through 14 abstinent months of smoldering anger, exploding in rage. But that anger had a much longer history and Hal knew it. He tells us that he pushed himself to dig up the past too fast and too soon in recovery. He didn't have the time sober or the solidity of longer-term recovery to hold all the feelings.

This is often a difficult, unclear question for the patient and the therapist: how much to facilitate opening up memories of the past and the emergence and expression of affect? Once again, the therapist follows the patient closely, being careful not to impose the therapist's preferred theory or modality, independent of an understanding of this particular patient. Many therapists believe that helping a patient feel is always desirable, an axiom about what constitutes good therapy. This is simply not true. If Hal was maintaining abstinence without much emotional turmoil and the process of recovery was in place and underway, the focus could stay in the present, on Hal and his building recovery. If Hal was not able to maintain abstinence and/or if he continued to experience intense psychological pain, we would look to other issues in the present such as his relationship with his wife, and his history, as the source of his current difficulties in stabilizing his abstinence and recovery.

This is one of the most controversial, no-right-answer-fits-all issues that may divide mental health and chemical dependence treatment teams. The therapist must be guided by a focus on alcohol and recovery, coupled with solid knowledge and skill in behavioral, cognitive, psychodynamic (including trauma), and systems theories. Most importantly, therapy should not be molded to fit the therapist's ideal of what good therapy should "look" like. "Good" therapy involves following the patient closely and knowing what constitutes "normal" recovery. It is not a preferred modality.

As it turned out for Hal and Maggie, neither one is sorry the explosion of rage occurred, as we see when the interviewer asks what their relationship is like now:

MAGGIE: Better. The anger was another bottom. It helped me set a boundary. I had let him run my life, but not anymore. This was a turning point for me and who I am. I stopped caring about his anger and began to care about myself. We started to talk together again. We have a long way to go.

In our first year we had a relationship. We talked, but it didn't match my fantasy of closeness. It wasn't bad. I was giving a lot and not getting. I was depressed but learning to take care of myself. When he was drinking I felt he could feel and care. He lost it with abstinence and I lost him.

This is not uncommon. The partner, who may be very pleased with abstinence, feels a loss of the alcoholic spouse emotionally. Many report that the alcoholic was more engaged, more accessible, and even more fun when drinking. It may take a long time in recovery for the alcoholic to become available again, or for the first time. Many partners will also discover that they too were not emotionally open or capable of mature relationship, an insight that usually comes as a complete surprise.

HAL: In those first months, some things were familiar and comfortable for us. But we weren't on to something new. Since I walked out, we've been on a different path. We're charting new turf. And we're intensely together on this road.

MAGGIE: We went to a workshop a few months into recovery. I didn't want to go because I was afraid to open anything up. But I realized he was going down a recovery path and I'd be left behind if I didn't get a program for myself. I tried to focus on myself. He said he was going to the workshop and I could come or not. It was an ultimatum about us.

HAL: I was setting priorities. I have to choose recovery over my marriage and anything else.

MAGGIE: Now we are separate and we have to respect our individuality. Before, I saw myself supporting him. Now I am focusing on myself.

When Maggie began to focus on herself, she could turn her attention away from what she wanted from Hal. At this point in Early Recovery, Maggie's shift in focus onto herself was a positive change that altered the system, breaking up what had been a drinking enmeshment that continued for her in recovery. Like Hal, she was also setting a foundation for a recovery process built on differentiation and a value of greater individual autonomy (Bader & Pearson, 1988).

HAL: I don't know where we are going. I'm not in control, but I have a better feeling about us. I was making major changes in my life and she was resisting. She wanted me to give her attention, and I wanted her to do it for herself. I felt afraid for my own recovery, but I don't now.

Hal moves to the past again as he remembers his parents:

HAL: My mother and father were both alcoholics. They would drink, fight, and pass out. The house went from chaos to silence. Then my father began to go to bars. I was with him, and he would drive on the wrong side of the street, off the road and even on to the sidewalk. It scared me to death. I can feel it now. There was a smell of fear in that car.

    When I was a teenager, my parents stopped drinking. Just like that. But absolutely nothing changed. They didn't go to AA, and they didn't get any help. They both got more silent and depressed. In a few years they got a divorce.

Listening, we realize that Hal needed Maggie to be in recovery herself and to be active, so he could have a partner rather than someone like his mother and father who "did nothing." Hal did not want Maggie controlling him, watching over him, and sacrificing herself either, which is how she saw her role in the couple relationship during the first year. For Hal, this was just too much like his mother. In a clinical setting, we might offer this interpretation.

    We hear issues of childhood trauma—living with out-of-control alcoholic parents. We also hear Hal speaking as an adult. If Hal had not been sober, we might include a focus on his past, but now we stay in the present. Hal tells us that he will be different than his parents were after they stopped drinking, which we sense is perhaps his strongest motivation at this time.

    The interview continues, and we ask about decision making:

MAGGIE: We talk more now, but if we disagree, we're in trouble. It's all or none. But I have hope that we can learn to communicate.

Now we are still more emotional than rational. We need professional help to talk with each other, as we can't make it up from
nothing.

Maggie illustrates the concrete level of thinking and feeling
common to Transition and Early Recovery. It is very difficult for
couples to build a dialogue together because it is still so hard to
understand and integrate ambiguity, more than one feeling or idea at
a time, and multiple layers of complexity that are part of a mature
relationship. Couples may also be impatient for solutions that may
temporarily solve a problem, but stifle openness to an ongoing process.

HAL: Decision making used to depend on whether it affected my
drinking. Now I can consider what I want, need, and feel.

The interviewer now asks if Hal and Maggie saw stages in their
recovery.

HAL: The first year was one stage—I went into treatment and recovery.
One year later I was grounded enough that she could collapse.
She always deferred her needs to mine. At 14 months we had a
crisis. Instead of detachment we had intense overinvolvement, I
exploded in rage, and we came crashing into each other. We had
been two people who always had a chemical buffer between us:
take alcohol away and something's gotta give.

MAGGIE: At first my focus was on him and alcohol. He had always
been "the patient," the one who got the attention. Only when he
was healthier could I collapse. After the alcohol's gone, there's a
stage of becoming independent—from the dependence on alcohol. He did that. I had to do it too, but I didn't realize it. I had
to give up my dependence on him, which I couldn't even see. It's
like adolescence: stormy. The crisis of rage was a turning point:
do we want to try to save this marriage.

Maggie describes the vacuum in self and relationship that follows
abstinence.

MAGGIE: The first year I didn't see that I needed help. I didn't see
myself as codependent. Now I see how I let other people decide
for me. In the first 7 months of his recovery I had to deal with

the death of my father and I had to deal with it by myself. He was not available.

We learn that Maggie was hurt and angry at the absence of support from Hal. She carried these feelings and her jealousy of his involvement in AA for a long time, which, we think, probably contributed to her resistance to seeing herself as a "codependent," a partner in the drinking or recovery system.

HAL: Maggie refused to call herself codependent, which made me angry. I was tired of being the identified patient, the one with all the problems. They're not just my problems.

MAGGIE: In the first year I focused on him and I was standing still. I started to crawl and then to walk after the first year. I changed my attitude toward myself and focused on myself. But I couldn't do this without getting help.

Here we see evidence of one of our core principles: members of the couple need to reach outside the system for help.

HAL: We created a crisis between us. I think subconsciously we knew we could do it, that we had to open up the difficult stuff. It wasn't conscious though, so it was chaotic, emotional, and out of control. Before this, we had tried to manage our relationship in a rational way. This scared us, and woke us up.

Psychologically minded, with a past history of therapy, Hal has insight about his explosion of anger. While Hal and Maggie see it as an opportunity for positive growth and change—they use it to shatter the status quo—others might feel more frightened and seek additional support to contain the feelings. AA and Al-Anon members might increase their meetings and emphasize the 12 steps to help them understand their core issues and motivations, and to contain deeper feelings. Some might fear that such an expression of affect would lead to a relapse, which indeed it might, so they postpone any exploration at all. Others might conclude that suppressing expression of feeling and tabling exploration might lead to a relapse. Clearly, there is not one correct course. Hal and Maggie opened the feelings. Hal increased his attendance at AA meetings, and Maggie started Al-Anon.

We ask who had been the most meaningful person to each of

them. Maggie says it was her therapist, and Hal says: "Me. I have found my self. I never had a sense of self that was mine, that couldn't be crossed. I never realized I could have myself until recovery. Now I realize it has to be for me and it is life or death."

Hal is passionate about recovery and his need to find himself.

HAL: When I was drinking, I didn't have a separate identity, though I tried to find it in drinking. At the beginning of recovery, I would have lived alone if I could have recognized that I had a choice. Maggie saw herself as supporting me, which became a huge burden to me.

Hal grasps that recovery is a process. Being in recovery has an impact on him that alters his experience of himself, which then changes his views and experience of recovery. Hal says that it's an interaction. Philosophically, he says he and Maggie have to take action, to risk being actively involved in creating their lives. Otherwise, a passive replaying of his own childhood and his deep identification with his parents will be his destiny. From a psychodynamic perspective we can guess that his passion and drive for action are fueled in part by his fear of repeating his parents' "do nothing, change nothing" passivity when they stopped drinking, as well as his fear of depression.

Toward the end, we ask if they have a family story of recovery. Maggie indicates her growth as she acknowledges that they are both recovering individuals as well as a couple. But she also defers to Hal, which is what upset him early on.

MAGGIE: We are members of a couple, and we are recovering individuals. Hal still pushes change, and I follow. I had no role in his seeking recovery, and it's hard for me to initiate change now.

Hal emphasizes the critical crisis they have just been through. He lays it out: they both have to be involved in recovery—a joint venture—or they will not change.

HAL: Whose recovery are we talking about? Nine months ago I was the patient. Now we've each got a part. I'm the mover, the driver, the one most likely to take the leap first. "Writing" a family story is something we do together. I'm the one who raises issues, but

Maggie joins right away. We interact with each other and recovery, and our story changes. It's not static. The story holds us and our lives. If we don't change, the story won't change either. When the curtain comes down, we will have lived out someone else's destiny. Now we have a chance to find ourselves and do it differently.

In our recovery check with the Turners, we see that they are in a new period of vulnerability, having "hit bottom" together just 2 months ago with an explosion of rage. The environment is tense, just like new abstinence. The system is in a sudden collapse, the kind of collapse the Turners did not experience when Hal stopped drinking. We assess their individual programs of recovery concretely: Are they both going to 12-step meetings regularly? (Maggie has just started going to Al-Anon.) Do they feel comfortable, do they share, do they each have a sponsor? If the answers are "No," we ask "Why?" Is there a problem or not? What about therapists? They have both had individual therapy in the past, and several ACOA therapy workshops in abstinence. Is this a time for adding therapy? Hal mentioned his mother and father several times and his childhood, so we consider the benefit of a more psychodynamic therapy for him at this time. We also pay close attention to his recent emotional experience of loss of control, being careful to emphasize containment of impulse, through a solid AA program, before facilitating uncovering therapy. Hal told us he opened up too much too soon, even though neither he nor Maggie are sorry. However, we do not want to push for the same quick exploration and expression of affect. First, we determine that structures of abstinence are in place; next, that people can use them; and only then do we support a focus on childhood and an uncovering therapy.

At less than 2 years of abstinence, we know that relapse is still common and therefore Hal is at significant risk. As years are accrued in recovery, relapse is less common. But it can occur *at any time* for *any person*. Thus, we *never* fail to assess the strength or weakness of the recovery program. All therapeutic interpretations and interventions at any point in time are made with consideration of the rock-bottom importance of abstinence.

CHAPTER FOUR

From Early Recovery to Ongoing Recovery

THE HENDERSONS AND THE WARNERS

THE HENDERSONS: 5 YEARS' ABSTINENCE— INTO ONGOING RECOVERY

The Hendersons, Patsy (44) and Roger (46), live in a small Southern California community with their sons John (14) and Eddie (12), and their daughter, Trish (17). Patsy and Roger each have 5 years of abstinence from alcohol, and both have attended AA regularly during the entire period. Their sons participated in the interview for the first half hour.

This is a family thoroughly saturated and organized by alcohol during the drinking and equally organized by alcohol—that is, recovery—now. What is it like with two alcoholic parents who stop drinking and begin recovery at the same time? We will see that the Hendersons have a stable, secure environment and recovery system at 5 years of abstinence. They illustrate how both reached outside the family at the point of abstinence, relinquishing reliance and dependence on the other, to focus separately on their individual recoveries. Reliance on AA and their sponsors allowed their old family system to stay in collapse and the building of a new, healthy system to evolve as a result of healthy individual development.

Initially, in the interview, we ask the children about themselves:

what they like best in school, and least; where they go on vacation and if they like it. Then we turn our attention to alcoholism. We want to get a sense of how both parents' recoveries influence and organize the family now. With 5 years of abstinence, would we see a stable environment and a changed family system? How would the children think about alcoholism and recovery? So we start with a focus on the present, rather than the past.

ROGER: Our alcoholism and recovery are a part of normal family life. So it's not different, unusual, or something we talk about.

PATSY: We've got alcoholics coming through the house all the time, and the kids ask us if that's a new "baby." We've traveled a lot with Roger's work, so they've been to meetings all over the world.

ROGER: But it's rare for us to have a conversation about a particular meeting. I go to over 500 AA meetings a year, so it's just a normal, significant part of life. I often go to noon meetings, as it's a nice break from the office.

PATSY: Our lives are very busy. We're both involved with school and sports activities—Roger coaches the soccer team. We're outgoing and entertain a lot. The kids have had a lot of close relationships with sober alcoholics, and they've gone to lots of meetings.

We immediately notice the ease between Patsy and Roger as they respond directly to us while maintaining a dialogue together. They demonstrate an ability and a freedom to speak for themselves as individuals, at the same time collaborating to tell us a family story. We turn to the kids and ask, "What do we need to know about you and your family?" Without a blink, John answers so clearly we have no doubt what counts: his parents show up for him.

JOHN: My parents come to every game. The whole family comes, even Grandpa. I have an uncle who lives nearby, and he comes too when he's in recovery. I don't remember too much about their drinking. I used to get beers for my dad when we'd watch football.

   It's not important to me that my parents are in recovery. It is important that they go to meetings.

INTERVIEWER: What do you think about the fact that your parents are alcoholics?

JOHN: Are they weird, you mean? No, this is normal. My parents can leave home pissed off, go to a meeting, and come home feeling good. It's normal for parents to go to meetings.

EDDIE: I came prepared for this question. It's not weird. They seem like normal parents, just like my friends' folks.

John and Eddie talk more about everyday life. John is worried about a friend whose actively alcoholic father is physically abusing him. John offers support and suggestions for how his friend might cope. Then the children leave the interview and we proceed with the parents.

INTERVIEWER: What was it like during the drinking?

ROGER: Drinking was my solution. I was screwed up and drinking solved it. By the time I was in college people were telling me to go to AA.

PATSY: I went to everything for my kids. I thought I was overcompensating for his behavior. The kids had care, from one parent at a time. He drove them when I was too hung over. In recovery we both worked with good sponsors who told us to always focus on our own recovery. They wouldn't let us get involved with each other's programs the way we covered for each other's drinking. Roger got the Al-Anon message to give me unconditional love and let go—that my life was none of his business. He got a travel job after a few months, which gave me more space. We couldn't afford to separate, though we needed to. We were joined at the hip. It took AA and our sponsors to get us to separate.

This early sobriety was the first time either of us had ever had a sense of separateness in any relationship. We went to our first two meetings together, and then we only went to meetings together on the weekends. Now it doesn't matter as much.

We were incapable of talking about it at all in the beginning. It was overwhelming. We both talked with our sponsors, and that was draining.

Patsy and Roger illustrate how outside sources of help facilitated the collapse of their enmeshed drinking system while facilitating differentiation between them. Their sponsors told them to attend different AA meetings, thus indirectly encouraging their physical and emotional "separation." People in AA will likely give the same advice to all newcomers: focus on yourself, and let your partner do the same. This focus on the self, along with attendance at AA and Al-Anon—as individuals—facilitates the breakup of unhealthy dependent relationships (Brown, 1988, 1993). Working the 12 steps, with a focus on the self, interrupts the defenses that maintain interpersonal pathology, including denial, projection, externalization, and rationalization.

This advice, to focus on the self, is a neutral systems intervention. It is not a directive to reject or abandon one's partner, although that is how it may feel to both. The universality and neutrality of this advice help soften the sudden interruption to the unhealthy drinking partnership.

INTERVIEWER: What was family life like?

ROGER: We didn't get meals before. The kids were lucky if they got breakfast.

PATSY: They were "alcoholic self-sufficient" kids. When I sobered up and looked in the refrigerator there was nothing there but pizza cartons and Chinese food. I always thought it was because of barbecue season. It was because I was an alcoholic. We were affluent, but we neglected our kids.

We came into recovery the first time 9 years ago, and they saw it all. When we started drinking again, we hid it. I used to be hung over and yell a lot. Eddie's teacher called one time to see if there were family problems. Another time he set off the burglar alarm so the police would come. If I had been a lower-bottom alcoholic, they might have taken my kids from me, but we lived in a nice home in a nice neighborhood.

Patsy knows that she and Roger were protected by their affluence from some of the consequences of child neglect and endangerment. Patsy paints a shocking picture of reality. Living with parental alcoholism is traumatic for kids. She also illustrates her "skewed" alcoholic reasoning. There was an explanation for this reality that normalized it—barbecue season—and the problem was gone.

PATSY: In early recovery we didn't leave the kids alone. Others told us they'd survive, but I disagreed. They were 7, 9, and 12 years old then.

In recovery they paid attention to their kids immediately. This care and protection are essential for all children, though it is often very difficult for parents to achieve early on, emotionally or logistically.

Asked what changes occurred over the next 2–5 years, Patsy and Roger fill in their portrait of Early Recovery. They describe a disorganized, chaotic, out-of-control home life, which continued for several years. This was similar to the drinking, except all the chaos was about recovery: the dramatic changes the family makes and the changes they must accommodate to. Although they both eagerly embraced AA and went to meetings every day, the next 4 years were difficult, particularly for Patsy.

PATSY: It was easy to see the changes with Roger. It was like night and day in his reactions to the kids. I was nuts for 2 years and was still not good the third year. I had an alcoholic father. Neither my mother or father was interested in our recoveries—being alcoholic and being sober didn't mean anything to them. In fact, it threatened them. It was very hard. My mother died when I had 13 months of sobriety.

Here we again see the generational nature and influence of alcoholism. Patsy had an alcoholic father, who, along with her mother, could not be supportive of her when she stopped drinking. It simply was too threatening for them. Recovery for ACOAs like Patsy often brings deep loss. Recovery may mean disloyalty and the breaking of family ties. It was extremely difficult for Patsy to be in recovery and lose her bond to her parents because of it.

PATSY: I felt chaos and was always asking myself, "Can I take one more thing?" We couldn't do sex sober. I had a big withdrawal and a lot of fear. I didn't know what to do. It took a long time for our sex life to become normal. When it did we joked about whether to call our sponsors and tell them.

As an alcoholic woman I was sexual. Sobered up, I was the Virgin Mary. I had to actually start making love for that to go away. If you've only done something drinking, you can't do it sober. It felt abnormal to have sex, and all feelings felt strange. This was hard for us because we didn't have any sexual problems when we were drinking.

Patsy illustrates the new, unknown terrain of abstinence. People have to learn everything over, minus alcohol, which is a great shock. What was automatic and associated with alcohol, like sex, is awkward and unnatural without it.

ROGER: Patsy was nuts for the first 3 or 4 years. We both stopped smoking, and I had some surgeries. I was depressed a lot of the time.

John and Eddie enter the room briefly to check in. There is an easy exchange of information, focused on what the kids have done so far and what they will do for the remainder of the interview. Again we note the openness between everyone and the parents' ability to pay attention to their children in the moment. When the kids leave, Patsy recalls how dominated by alcohol her life, and thus her children's lives, had been:

PATSY: The kids are very aware of recovery, and they are antidrug now. But I don't think they'd be sober if we hadn't stopped. I always thought of myself as a social drinker. I liked the sophistication of it, and I always had a capacity to drink. I had a history of picking alcoholic men—two husbands—who abused me. In all our family pictures I had a drink in my hand.

With this description, Patsy illustrates how thoroughly she and her world were dominated by chronic alcoholism, despite the fact that she thought of herself as a social drinker.

With 5 years of abstinence, Patsy and Roger have a history of recovery to tell us, with as much growth and change as the downward progression of their drinking. Not only are they attentive, involved parents; they also demonstrate a much more equal couple relationship. They can discuss issues or problems in an open, exploratory way without having to prematurely draw conclusions to end the anxiety of open-ended dialogue. When the interviewer asked how decision making has changed, Patsy and Roger illustrate a hallmark of mature communication: reciprocity. Dialogue is a real conversation—back and forth.

ROGER: Before, in making decisions, we did it my way. She could comment or not. Now, we express our opinions and differences. Before I would have kept quiet. She always did the financial end.

In recovery I wanted to be involved, and at first she was annoyed. None of these changes came easily. Now we have family meetings regularly to plan everything.

INTERVIEWER: So you have discussions?

ROGER: Our process is amiable, though there is some tension. We don't argue or fight, though we do disagree. Neither one of us has trouble expressing anger, though I might stuff it. We used to fight all the time when we were drinking.

PATSY: Roger expresses his anger, and he's done with it. I carry it around.

ROGER: But it's not a "big deal" kind of anger now.

PATSY: We do irritation and quick anger.

In describing the way they deal with anger, Patsy and Roger illustrate maturity individually and as a couple. They know what they feel and what they do with feelings. Anger is not taboo, and it is not buried. It is also not the currency of exchange, as it was during drinking, not the link to engagement and intimacy—a false intimacy, of course. We sense openness and flexibility between them, which will lead to closeness.

INTERVIEWER: What is recovery like now?

PATSY: We are stable, and our growth is slower. Other crises are resolved, and we don't see the kind of radical growth now that we had in the beginning.

ROGER: It was explosive growth to begin with and then a leveling. We've come together closer than ever as a result of separating.

PATSY: He used to track my drinking, and I felt like a hostage.

ROGER: As I developed as an individual, I was able to let her be who she is. If I want a good marriage, I'd better be a whole person, not just a half.

PATSY: We live well together.

We then ask if they have a shared, family story.

PATSY: Yes, and also separate. He always sees that things are going well in recovery, and I wonder if we're living in the same house.

ROGER: We often have two different stories about the same thing.

In this segment, they emphasize the process of separating emotionally and the intense focus on individual growth during Early Recovery. They illustrate a humorous acceptance of differences, a hallmark of healthy relationship.

Finally we asked who had been the most meaningful person to each of them in recovery?

ROGER: My sponsor.

PATSY: My sponsor. We both got sponsors within 3 or 4 days, and they knew what to do. We focused on ourselves and on sober people. We let go of our drinking friends. It was hard for us early on because we didn't know any couples who were both in recovery. We have seen that many couples get divorced if only one of them is in recovery.

Here we see evidence of our core finding: the critical importance of the collapse of the drinking system, a systemic alteration that is maintained by seeking help outside of the family. Both of these factors facilitate emotional separation and the interruption of unhealthy relational dependence.

In our recovery check we see that the Hendersons are what we might call an AA couple through and through. The environment is safe, secure, consistent, and predictable. The Hendersons have a new family system organized around alcoholism recovery, and they are committed to their individual recoveries. We assess for holes, as always, past and present therapies (data that we collected from everyone in the demographic questionnaire), and the need for any changes, modifications, or intervention now. A few weeks after the interview, Patsy called asking for a referral for individual therapy. The process of the interview opened up painful memories of her childhood and abusive marriages that she wanted to address.

THE WARNERS: 13 YEARS' ABSTINENCE—
ONGOING RECOVERY

The Warners, Kay (49), and Randy (54) and two of their four children, Sonia (32) and Barry (30), participated in the interview in Palo Alto, California. Kay has been abstinent for 13 years in AA, and she has also been in therapy. Sonia has been sober for 14 years with AA and therapy, and Barry has been clean of alcohol and other drugs for 5 years, also with AA, therapy, and a recovery-oriented church. One other child is sober, and the fourth is not an alcoholic, according to everyone. Randy has been in Al-Anon, a 12-step ACOA program, and therapy.

The interviewer asked what it was like during the drinking. As you'll see, the Warners have a story of active alcoholism and recovery that includes each individual and the family as a whole. They remember clearly what it was like, but they also have many years in recovery with a lot of difficult times, good times, and deep changes to tell us about. They are an example of a mentor family in Ongoing Recovery.

KAY: There was a lot of insanity. I wanted to escape emotionally so I would not feel or care. I was a binge drinker, so I never knew where it would take me. I drank to the point I didn't think about anything. I would lose time and be in a blackout all the time.

I drank before my marriage, and then I stopped when I was having children. When the youngest child was 8 months old I started drinking again. Then I started working in a bar. In that atmosphere I felt free. I had no responsibilities, and I wanted to stay in that frame of mind and not come back to reality. I drank nights at the bar and never at home. He took care of the kids at night. I led two separate lives.

The atmosphere was insane, but I couldn't see it. I had no idea. One time Barry was in trouble at school—for acting out—and they wanted us to come in for a family meeting. There was no way I was going to that meeting. All of our kids acted out: three of the four became alcoholics.

Kay describes the drinking, defensive "false self." She was driven by internal chaos, which she re-created in her life. She describes the impact of her out-of-control double identity and chaotic double lives. Her kids responded to her drinking and the "insane" atmosphere by doing the same thing: drinking and "acting out." The day-to-day norm was chaos and out-of-control behavior, which becomes stabilized, chronic trauma (Brown, 1994).

SONIA: I became responsible and I hated Mom. I knew something was wrong, that it wasn't normal, but I thought if I was good enough and kept the house clean there would be no problem. But I knew it was alcohol. I went to Al-Anon at 11 and 12, but I got into trouble with Mom and that was the end of that. I hung out with older kids, and when I got a drink down me it was magic.

I was angry and afraid all the time. I was afraid to tell my opinion, so I was quiet. When I drank I was everything I wanted to be. I could do anything! But I was going to blow up with everything inside of me I couldn't tell.

So I became a problem and I drank (at 15). I tried to get along with my mother—we went barhopping. It was all we could do together. I drove her.

Sonia illustrates the impact on her of living with trauma: the fear, anger, need to "tell," and her inability to tell. She describes what trauma theorists (van der Kolk, McFarlane, & Weisaeth, 1996; Herman, 1992) call "traumatic bonding," the securing of attachment through pathology. Sonia says the only thing she could do with her mother was drink with her and drive her to bars.

SONIA: One day I got up and looked in the mirror: I had turned into what I didn't want to be. I didn't want to wake up. I took pills and threw up. Then one day I wanted to live. I called AA and I went. I was 18, and I haven't had a drink since.

BARRY: I didn't know why Mom was sick all the time. She was always in bed, hung over. I finally realized: Mom comes home in different moods and takes it out on everyone. All the kids were in a shell. I got away with a lot. I drove cars really young; I stole. I loved to get into trouble, into fights. I did what I was supposed to. At 16 I realized that Mom had a problem with alcohol. I just kept doin' what I was doin'.

What does Barry mean: "I did what I was supposed to"? We surmise that he was expressing—behaviorally—family realities that could not be acknowledged or spoken about, imitating and modeling (Brown, 1988) his mother's behavior, and calling attention to the family chaos at the same time. We will learn later that Kay's drinking and her chaotic lifestyle were related to avoiding recognition of her alcoholic parents and of being molested as a child. The same will be true for Barry.

And last, Randy remembers. Like the others, he focuses on himself: what it was like for him, how he thought, and what he did. He tells us how he tried to make sense of things that made no sense and how he tried to cope:

RANDY: Life was chaotic. Kay was pregnant when we married, and we had four kids in 4 years. I felt sorry for her, so I worked two jobs and let her spend. In a few years we were in bankruptcy. So she got the job in the bar. I was against it at first, and it got worse. She was out all night. But I grew up in an alcoholic family. You had to put up with things. This is the way it was.

Randy's internal experience—his "idea"—of family life was chaos and drinking, exactly what he and Kay created unconsciously.

RANDY: Sonia came to me and cried. I consoled her. Kay and I were so young, and we knew so little. It was hard to get feedback about what we were doing wrong, and it was hard keepin' things together. Sometimes she wanted a divorce, she wanted to throw me out because I didn't stop her.
    I wasn't open then. I always acted, and she screamed. I punished the kids—whatever had to be done.

Randy illustrates a paradoxical dilemma about control. He knew something was terribly wrong for his wife and for him, but he had no idea what to do about it. He tried to do more of the same, which for him was to work harder, in order to gain a feeling of control himself. Although such efforts to achieve more control may seem to make logical sense, they tend to produce the opposite effect: more chaos and more loss of control in the environment, in the family drinking system, and for all individuals within it.

KAY: We got a house with the idea of helping the kids. I didn't drink for a couple of months, and then I stayed drunk. I was afraid of everything. I did this for 6 months. I called Sonia; she'd been sober already so she told me she wouldn't pick me up anymore. I wanted to kill her. I slammed the phone. I saw the change in her. She wasn't depressed; I saw the freedom in her eyes. We were no support to her then.
    One day I had a "moment of clarity" and I knew alcohol was

my problem. I called Sonia and asked her to take me to an AA meeting, and I got real involved.

This is Kay's point of surrender, of hitting bottom and asking for help.

SONIA: All I ever wanted was for Mom to get sober and give me a hug. We had plenty of material things, but it was hard to stay sober at first. I had to let go of my family and of thinking I could do anything to make my mother happy and sober. When I gave up trying, she called. She did it for herself. The healing started. We were able to tell each other the way we felt and to make amends the best we could. We started our relationship from there.

Here Sonia emphasizes the relationship with her mother, which was organized around alcohol. She also illustrates the break in her alcoholic attachment: "I had to let go of my family and give up trying to make my mother happy."

Randy tells us how tuned out he was to all the chaos. Soon, he will tell us what it took and how long it took for him to get "tuned in."

RANDY: I don't remember a lot. I was a commuting workalcoholic, gone weeks at a time.

INTERVIEWER: Did you notice when Sonia quit drinking?

RANDY: Yes, but I didn't give it a lot of attention. I didn't know anything. That's why I worked all the time.

BARRY: I didn't see a lot. I was mad, and I was still using [alcohol and other drugs]. I thought, "They're all gonna get sober and I'm not"; they were a threat to me. I had to go to prison first.

KAY: In Early Sobriety there was an awful lot of insanity. It was still hard to deal with anything because I didn't have the tools and skills. It was hard to cope sober with the kids acting out, and I didn't have any support from Randy. I didn't get into therapy for 5 years.

We hear mention of denial, avoidance. Randy and Barry didn't see, didn't pay attention. Kay says, "It was insane early on." She was sober, but she had no tools. There was a vacuum without alcohol and nothing to replace it. It was a major turning point when Randy and Kay assumed a parental role and added structure to the family system. They established rules that became a foundation for a new healthy family system.

KAY: We ended up having house rules. Everyone had to come into the house at a decent time and had to be clean and sober. No substances [alcohol and other addictive and intoxicating drugs] could come into the house. The kids had to pay rent. We kicked two of the kids out for breaking the rules.

In Transition and Early Recovery therapists are tracking the vacuum, staying abreast as to how family members are filling it or not, and assessing the need for additional structure. This family lived in a chaotic environment and a destabilized system for at least 5 years. Then, a crisis moved the family to another level of recovery.

KAY: At 5 years I got cancer, went into therapy, and Barry went to prison.

RANDY: It was a turning point for me. My boss said I was fired if I missed work to be at the hospital with Kay. I knew then how important she was and that life was too short to lose her.

KAY: Everyone made drastic changes then. Till that time [therapy] I had no clue that my molestation as a child had anything to do with my emotional problems. I started ACOA work and focused on that for the next 4 years.

Before that, in the beginning of sobriety, I got very involved with AA. In my fourth year I got real depressed, did more inventories, and had a good sponsor. I did everything I was told, and it wasn't working. I got scared and wasn't sure I wanted to be sober. I said, "If this is all there is, it's not enough." Then I found out I had cancer.

There was more for me. I just didn't know it. Being sober was good enough for a while, and then it wasn't. With therapy a whole new world opened up and everything made sense.

Kay illustrates the layered development of individual and family recovery. For the first 5 years, the focus was on individual growth, outside the family through AA and Al-Anon. At 5 years, the family was stabilized enough in abstinence to allow another "hitting bottom," with a systems collapse, to occur. The Warner family then embarked on a second process of destabilization and growth, organized on a foundation of recovery. Now, the focus was on the past, opening up ACOA and trauma issues for at least two generations.

We see that the first tier of recovery was focused on cognitive–behavioral change to maintain abstinence and a gradual reduction in chaos and out-of-control behavior. The second tier emphasized psychodynamic work to open up the past. This depth of individual uncovering would not have been possible without the foundation of abstinence to contain and structure the emerging memories and affect.

KAY: All of our lives are so different today. It seems like a story. We have no secrets today. We talk about everything. What was so sick—the secrets and the lies. We always minimized how bad things were.

Kay illustrates how much she and others tried to hold things together; but it didn't work. There were still secrets and lies that had to come out:

BARRY: I was molested by my cousin till I went to prison. We referred to it as "the issue." I turned 21 in prison. I used to go out to speak at AA and with the prison guards.

KAY: We visited Barry in prison once a month and did a lot of healing in there. I had the same anger and rage then as Barry. I didn't know yet that he was an incest survivor.

I learned about molestation. Everyone minimized it. I tried to talk about it, and people got angry. They asked me why would I go to ACOA with so much sobriety? Why would I go back in time? It was hard because I wanted their approval. But the nightmares started, I got into therapy, and the memories came.

Sonia tells us what a hard time this was. Her mother had resisted opening up, and everyone in the family resisted too.

SONIA: I tried to be supportive of Mom in therapy. But the more therapy she had, the more moody and depressed she got. I had a sour taste on therapy because she was worse off.

I didn't understand. Then I did; she was goin' back and clearin' up the stuff. But it was hard. I kept wondering why she'd put herself in so much pain living in the past.

KAY: Everybody said that. I got no validation.

RANDY: Kay told me we had to go to therapy to stay together. I needed it too.

KAY: I knew we had to grow together or we'd grow apart.

RANDY: I was resistant, and yet I wanted to support her. It was very hard for me. I'm glad we did it now. We had couples and individual therapy.

BARRY: My mom sent me a *Big Book* and a *Twelve By Twelve* in prison. I started to go to meetings. One time our whole family was in therapy together and everybody, including the spouses, was in recovery. We had a lot of neat experiences. Before, we lived in a house full of strangers.

In this family no one was left out. Over 14 years each person "crossed over," joining the increasingly stronger recovery core. The family now, like night and day, evolved and grew, building on its own base of change over many years.

SONIA: We used to beat each other up. There were holes in the walls and doors. If you got mad, you took that person out. We used to go to the park and pick fights for fun, just to get the anger out.

BARRY: We took karate lessons in recovery and got good at that.

KAY: God gave me a second chance with my grandchildren. They've never seen me drunk, in a rage, or hitting anybody. They're breaking the cycle.

This is an emotional moment. Kay summarizes it for everyone: they have been able to change; they don't have to pass it on. Then they talk about just how much they've changed as the interviewer asks about decision making.

KAY: A lot didn't change in the first 5 years. A lot of behaviors didn't change, and there was a lot of distance between us. After 5 years and therapy, we don't make a decision without talking it over.

RANDY: We share in delegating too.

Next the interviewer asks if they see themselves as an alcoholic family. Many of our families have trouble with this question. Some respond as if the idea of an "alcoholic family" nullifies the good and all the changes they have made. Others think the term must mean that someone is still drinking. Those who seem most comfortable with the words "alcoholic family" readily tell us how much recovery from alcoholism has organized their families now.

RANDY: We used to see ourselves as an alcoholic family. It's just a way of life now—without alcohol. We see ourselves as a recovering family if we think about it. It just keeps going on.

KAY: When people see us and hear what our lives were like, they can't believe it.

I just couldn't get enough at first. Now, I don't have to have so much; I don't have to run to a meeting. I have a circle of friends I talk to all the time. I have meetings on the phone. At first I had to have people in my life all the time, take care of people, sponsor others. Not so much now.

We hear a decrease in Kay's need for intensity and action, with the learning of Early Recovery now internalized.

SONIA: Drinking was our problem. We didn't know how to live. You take alcohol out, and what do you do now?

Like our other families, Sonia says there's a hole, a vacuum, when you take alcohol out. Initially, being in recovery fills the hole. Over time, recovery creates a foundation and the space for healthy development to flourish.

The interviewer then asks if family members can see stages in their recovery.

KAY: Yes, but they're hard to pinpoint. It's always evolving. I remember a fear of letting go of the person I thought I was—which was domineering. I kept wanting to keep a hold of part of that, or you'll be the hole in the doughnut. I was stepping out into something that's not there; no ground to stand on. It took me a couple of years. That was a stage.

That evolved to "guilt-ridden alcoholic mother." I had a lot of guilt. I was always playing make-up and catch-up. I was starting to realize what I'd done with my life and to see all I'd lost.

Up to the fourth year I was still pretty numb. I asked myself: Is this all there is to sobriety? The big event was getting into therapy. I was wondering what was wrong with me. I always thought everything was my fault. Then I saw that I had gloom and doom and no balance in my life. Now I'm trusting the process and change is coming.

RANDY: The first phase: she got into AA. Everyone ignored me, and it was all her. In therapy I saw a lot of the problem was me. I was an enabler, a people pleaser.

The second phase: she got cancer, which changed both our lives. It changed the way I thought about life. Now I live for the moment. I didn't want to lose her.

The third phase: Now I want to know what life is all about. What is the purpose? I also joined a men's group. I haven't had too many male friends, so I'm working on male bonding. My best friend had been my wife.

Kay and Randy illustrate beautifully what a developmental process of change is all about.

Finally, the interviewer brings the family to the end of their story so far, or at least to the end of telling it, with this question: "When was the whole family grounded in recovery?"

SONIA: When Barry was in prison we all went up there. We talk all the time about family. And every party, we make a big deal of it, which we never did before. After the party, we sit around and talk. "Wow, that was good! Nobody got in a fight, nobody got hit." We sibs all call each other and help each other. It's such a change from when Mom and Dad had scenes—like a cycle is changing with the rest of us. We're passing on recovery instead of the disease.

KAY: It's hard to be around other families now. You see the dysfunction.

SONIA: I don't like to be "inside" of it or involved.

KAY: The other two kids are changing too. Anna is a nurse, and Richie is a parole counselor. He got sober at 16.

SONIA: Our father was a "yes-man." We thought he was a wimp. We never knew anything about him. Now he has opinions, he shows emotion, and he's very affectionate with us and our kids. To watch the intimacy, to see the change, see him with the kids, is awesome.

Our recovery check yields a family portrait of a safe, secure environment, a healthy system, and healthy family relationships, with an ongoing process of dynamic individual growth and change. Kay has been free of cancer for seven years. This family has utilized outside supports, including 12-step programs and therapy, to maintain a dynamic process of growth for individuals and the family as a whole for 13 years. The Warners have a strong recovery.

PART THREE

A Framework for Assessment

CHAPTER FIVE

Assessing Family Functioning

DOMAINS OF EXPERIENCE

As we listened to the family's experiences in recovery, it became clear that different kinds of changes are occurring simultaneously on multiple levels. It is important and reassuring for families to be able to recognize the differences. Borrowing from prior research (Brown, 1991a, 1991b, 1991c, 1995a, 1995b) we listened with three theoretical frames, or domains, simultaneously in mind, along with the stage of recovery: the environment, the system, and individual development. Only by tracking movement on these multiple levels could we begin to understand the complexities of individual development and interpersonal interaction, both inherent to the process of family change. It is essential for therapists working with individuals, couples, and families to carefully assess each domain in order to pinpoint progress and difficulties more accurately. The source of problems may lie within a particular domain, or family members may be at different stages and thus have different needs. Assessing domains and stages helps determine the focus of what we referred to earlier as "next-step" concrete intervention—behavioral, cognitive, dynamic (including trauma) or systems.

We will review each of these domains now, highlighting family systems concepts that structured the way we listened to families and charted change. We will also suggest practical ways to add support to the family (and its individual members) during this time of radical change.

Our review of the three domains is a brief summary of theory. We refer therapists to the vast literature in each field for in-depth explication. Our purpose is not to teach readers these frameworks but to show therapists how to listen and think within these schemas, which are themselves controversial, with multiple points of view. We will continue to emphasize the importance of developmental theory, centered on loss of control, as the central organizing principle of recovery.

THE ENVIRONMENT

The environment refers to "what it was like": the experiences of daily, routine family life. It also includes the context of family life: who, where, what, when, plus the atmosphere, or "feel," of the home, and degrees of consistency and predictability and of chaos or order (Brown, 1991c, 1994). The environment holds the sense of basic security for all: Is this a safe place, emotionally and physically? Cary Corwin described her fear and the absence of safety with both her mother and father: "It was scary for me. We went from a good relationship and a solid safe place, which I counted on, to nothing."

Patsy Henderson described her children as "alcoholic self-sufficient. . . . We were affluent, but we neglected our kids."

Over the last decade it has been widely accepted that the alcoholic home environment is traumatic (Brown, 1988, 1991a, 1991b; Cermak, 1986; Black, 1981) which means that the individuals within the family feel a fundamental threat to their basic sense of self and well-being (Krystal, 1978; van der Kolk, 1987; van der Kolk et al., 1996; Terr, 1991; Herman, 1992). They may carry a feeling of chronic fear, even outright terror, and a need to be on guard (Brown, Beletsis, & Cermak, 1989). Families living with trauma often report that they feel unprotected and, as a result, insecure and frightened. Sonia Warner recalls that she was "angry and afraid all the time." Psychologists suggest that a feeling of internal and external safety is essential for establishing basic trust, the fundamental building block of healthy development (Erikson, 1963; Bowlby, 1988).

Most of our research families described the absence of emotional and physical safety living with chronic alcoholism, and especially as they approached the end of the drinking. One family said, "There was no trust. Nothing predictable. We couldn't plan anything. Family life was like a bad dream. Nothing to count on; nothing to hope for. We were all depressed."

An unsafe environment generates hypervigilant attention. The absence of safety sounds the alert for survival instincts and basic physical and emotional defenses (van der Kolk, 1987; van der Kolk et al., 1996). As one family said, "We had to be on guard. You just wait for some disaster."

The ongoing, normative experience of chaos, loss of control, and crisis reinforces and solidifies the need for defense as an adaptation. Then defense, in circular fashion, organizes the environment, the system, and individual development (Brown, 1988, 1995; Schmid, 1995). As one individual said:

> "Defense was all I had. Fighting off the horrible reality of drinking was all I could do. Denial took every ounce of energy. My view of myself, my family, had to fit in to my defended view of myself and everything else."

The therapist listens for and assesses context, the background and foreground of family life, which includes atmosphere, mood, tone, the kind and degree of chaos, and physical and emotional safety. This assessment of the environment informs the therapist's decisions about intervention: To what degree is the environment crisis dominated at this point in time? To what degree is everyone focused on reacting to and defending against the trauma of the environment? While a family is still drinking, and in the first weeks and months of abstinence, everyone's attention is geared toward safety and coping with the overwhelming chaos. The therapist may need to intervene aggressively in a dangerous situation, bringing in child protective services, for example, or moving family members out of the home. In another family, the therapist supports a child's view of reality and offers suggestions to help the child cope as adaptively as possible when the situation is not changing but when removal is not warranted or could make things worse for the child.

The therapist may help structure the priorities and activities of a newly recovering family, which quiets the chaos and fear. The Corwins, however, resisted anyone's efforts to help them deal with their hostile, unsafe environment. The atmosphere was full of anger, resentment, and resistance to being in recovery. Everyone could feel the overriding tension. Being open to recovery requires a vulnerability and willingness to suspend control that is impossible to maintain in such a hostile climate. In working with the Corwins, a therapist may note the state of crisis, tension, and hostility they have just described and wonder what is causing it. The therapist may also point out that no one is engaged in recovery. They are on hold. Why? What is in the way of the family moving into an attachment to recovery?

Other families can respond to help in creating more structure. Later, the environment becomes more predictable and stable, and attention shifts to the individuals within the family. The primary concern at the environmental level is safety—physical and emotional.

The involvement of an outsider allows the family to let go of control, which eventually leads to greater stabilization in the environment. Yet, in the worst of the chaos and calamity, family members are likely to try to exercise more control, in an effort to quiet the storm themselves. As one family said:

> "The harder we tried to hold it together, the worse it got. Our family therapist kept telling us we couldn't fix it by covering up so much and it wasn't going to go away. The therapist was right, but we didn't get it and we didn't like it."

The therapist helps the family tolerate the vacuum and chaos of new recovery by helping family members add structure and reassuring them that what they are experiencing is normal. The therapist also serves a protective function, watching for problems and making sure children are supervised and attended to. One therapist said,

> "I often give a minilecture on recovery. I tell the individual or family what to expect in recovery. I tell them the chaos is normal and explain how AA and Al-Anon meetings help each person, especially when they and the family aren't working yet. Sometimes I help families concretely, maybe working out a schedule. It's amazing how calming the schedule can be. When I work with them, it's easier to avoid the intense struggles that almost always characterize family interactions at this point. Many families can't talk and certainly can't agree on anything until much later. These are things a sponsor does too, but I am often involved before people get to 12-step meetings. Also, some family members are slower to go to 12-step meetings, or they never go. My explana-

tions help everyone feel heard and decrease some of the potential for family members to feel ignored and angry."

THE FAMILY SYSTEM

Family systems theory (von Bertalanffy, 1968; Watzlawick, Weakland, & Fisch, 1974; Bowen, 1974, 1978; Steinglass et al., 1987; Jacob, 1987; Bateson, 1971; Jacob, Dunn, & Leonard, 1981; Jacob, Favorini, Meisel, & Anderson, 1978; Gurman & Kniskern, 1981; Ackerman, 1958, 1994; Minuchin, 1992; Minuchin & Fishman, 1981; Minuchin, Montalvo, Guerney, Rosman, & Schumer, 1967) describes how the family works, the mechanisms or structure that allow it to function as a unit. The theory explains how interactional patterns of relationship and behavior maintain a family's sense of balance, or homeostasis. The theory suggests that all groups or families naturally strive toward achieving and maintaining internal stability, consistency, and cohesion.

This drive for balance locks the drinking family into its pathology. The same drive for stability, consistency, and cohesion can interfere with recovery. The family may be pulled back into the old patterns that give them a sense of familiarity and false security, rather than tolerating the chaos and uncertainty of early abstinence.

The foregoing statement is a central axiom that we will return to repeatedly as we describe the family's reactions to alcoholism. Its members efforts to cope and to keep the family intact often work, but they also make things worse. At the end of the line—the drinking line—when the family reaches recovery, many family members are still together. But in the process of staying intact *and* becoming an alcoholic family, everyone has given up some part, usually a big part, of his or her own healthy self. Becoming an alcoholic family requires an adjustment, at first a subtle tilting and then a radical turn, away from health, toward pathology. The power of people's need for others, for close relationship and sharing, outweighs and overrides their awareness of reality and the turn toward alcoholism that they are making. Not till much later, in recovery, can they look backward and chart the downward course that eroded everything (Steinglass et al., 1987; Treadway, 1989; Brown, 1985, 1988, 1995a).

In theory (Watzlawick et al., 1974), any change in one part of the system affects the entire family. These changes can be part of the normal developmental cycle of the family, such as the birth of a child or the departure of children for college or into marriage. They may also include important life events such as moving, illness, and perhaps recovery. The healthy family is not static. It maintains a fine, delicate balance that allows flexibility and fluidity for growth and change while never losing its internal stability. Just like a healthy person, the healthy family changes and grows while it remains recognizable and consistent.

The active alcoholic family is a system dominated by alcohol, alcoholism, or the alcoholic as the central organizing principle governing family dynamics and systems balance. As Maggie Turner said, "Alcohol was always the center of our relationship." The family grows in an unhealthy direction, becoming less fluid and flexible, more rigid and constricted, till no one can move. The family is arrested in development and may even be experienced as dying. The family in recovery is organized by a new process of growth that is grounded on abstinent principles and change.

With the Warner family we see consistent steps in systems change, beginning with Sonia's decision to stop drinking and go to AA. Kay followed, then Randy and Barry. As individuals moved into recovery one at a time, Kay and Randy strengthened the structure of the family by establishing clear rules and boundaries for a sober home. At 5 years of sobriety, Kay and Randy could focus on their relationship as a couple. Throughout their 13 years of abstinence, we see that the focus on the individual influenced the system and vice versa. Each family member needed to delve deeply within him- or herself, with a focus on the past and the present, in order for the parents and children to change and grow in a healthy direction as a family. That movement, in turn, paved the way for deeper individual growth.

Basic Systems Concepts

We will emphasize two major constructs of family systems theory: structure and process (Jacob, 1987). The therapist assesses both. In drinking, the structure is rigid and static because it is organized by pathology. With abstinence the structure collapses, making the absence of internal systems structure normal though very difficult. Attention has shifted to the individuals, away from the structural dominance of the pathological drinking system. Yet there may be gaps in structure that need attention immediately. Children need predictable schedules and routines even though the parents' lives may be in disarray. A therapist may also help with advice about family rules, roles, boundaries, and hierarchies in order to provide a temporary structure that will meet basic needs.

Process is ongoing. In the drinking family, it is reflecting, denying, and maintaining the pathology of alcoholism. In early abstinence, family process is focused on the individuals. Later, they can pay closer attention to the family directly, focusing on communication and interaction. The therapist monitors the normal process of recovery, alert to holes and ongoing resistance and problems.

Structure

Structure is the way the family is organized. It is also thought of as a "container" or "holder"—in essence, the bricks and mortar that give a particular "whole" its form. It includes five components: rules, roles, rituals, hierarchies, and boundaries (Jacob, 1987).

Rules. Rules are the stated and unstated guidelines for family function that become established and fortified by repetition. Because they express a family's core beliefs and values as well as a family's defenses, they may be unclear and even contradictory. With a drinking family, the therapist works toward making the underlying rules of deception and denial explicit. For example, over several sessions the therapist repeats, "In this family, everyone agrees not to talk about drinking."

In recovery, the therapist helps the family cope with the absence of rules and to avoid sliding back into old rules that no longer work. For example, the therapist says:

"It's hard to know what to do now that telling the truth is OK. It's all right not to know and to say so."

Healthy families have clear rules that are consistent with values and beliefs. But it takes a long time in recovery to get to this level of internal alignment.

The rule Kay and Randy Warner established—it was to be a dry home—reduced uncertainty and increased the safety everyone felt. The family members' beliefs about themselves and their recovery were now consistent with behavior. In drinking families unhealthy rules often support contradictions and secrets; for example, "It's OK to drink, but don't tell your mother."

*Roles.** Role is the function performed by someone or something in a familiar situation, process, or operation. Roles are expressed through repetitive behaviors and interactions with other family members. They can be healthy or unhealthy, either facilitating or interfering with positive family function. Roles have been part of the popular vocabulary in relation to alcoholic families for some time, including such terms as "caretaker," "placator," or "aggressor." In the Corwin family, Cary still has the role of worrying about, and even parenting, her father.

Role assignment is essential to any system. Knowing who belongs and who does what ensures stability, regardless of whether the roles are healthy. In the alcoholic family, the pattern of drinking behavior affects role assignment and stability. The nonalcoholic parent, if there is one, may regularly assume the roles and responsibilities of both father and mother, with the alcoholic parent incapacitated and excluded from the family's routine. The alcoholic may become another child, taken care of, cleaned up after, and not considered in decision making. Inconsistency may be minimal in such a home, although the inactive, childlike parent creates confusion for children. In later years, ACOAs commonly have difficulties with self-image and identity because they have not had appropriate healthy attachments or models. They are often dominated by defenses designed to overcome, mask, and undo pathogenic internalized models. ACOAs are likely to be afraid of repeating negative, destructive parental patterns.

In the drinking family, parents may change roles, depending on the drinking behavior of the alcoholic. Some alcoholics drink "periodically" or in a "binge" pattern that is alternated with periods of sobriety and stability. Their families adjust to the alternating patterns; all members are ready to switch roles when the alcoholic begins to drink.

Parents may take turns: one assumes responsibility while the other one drinks, and vice versa. Both parents present confusing and erratic models for their children and deprive them of predictable emotional

---

*The discussion of role assignment is adapted from Brown (1991c). Copyright 1991 by John Wiley & Sons, Inc. Adapted by permission.

availability. The consequences of the lack of any consistent, stable parental figure are severe.

In some alcoholic families, neither parent is competent and the child's attachment and relationship are characterized by role reversal. The child assumes a caretaking role with childlike, out-of-control parents. We saw this pattern with the Corwins, the Hendersons, and the Warners during drinking.

Rituals. Rituals are customs or family procedures that establish and maintain a family's identity and contribute to cohesiveness. In alcoholic families, important customs—birthdays, holidays, vacations—often become linked with drinking (Steinglass et al., 1987; Wolin, Bennett, & Noonan, 1979; Wolin & Bennett, 1984). As Cary Corwin reported, she came home from school and the whole family got "ripped" together. As we will illustrate later, it is extremely important to unhook family rituals from drinking and to establish new rituals that represent abstinence and new family values of recovery. Therapists can help directly by noting the value of rituals and perhaps helping the family think about what would be meaningful and appropriate to them. Sonia told us how the Warners shifted their enjoyment of wild parties to a positive family value. Their parties are now celebrated in the park, which used to be the place for violence: "You took that person out."

Hierarchies. Hierarchies are ordered subsystems within the family that are defined by function and task. For example, parents are at the top of the hierarchy and hold most of the responsibility for maintaining the family's survival. Frequently, the oldest child is next in line in terms of responsibilities, usually a mixed blessing. Problems can occur when the hierarchy shifts and/or when a child holds a position higher than a parent. This causes role confusion, improper balance of family power, and financial and emotional burdens.

With her father abstinent for 5 months, Cary Corwin is still functioning as a parent, a reversal of appropriate hierarchy as well as role. She is concerned about her father's lack of growth and change since he stopped drinking, evidenced by his anger, withdrawal and refusal to talk. Cary describes her continuing vigilance with her father: "I remember the sights and sounds, and I'm concerned when I'm not with him."

In drinking families, the relationship structure between the parents is usually unequal and polarized. The alcoholic is most often dominant, setting the rules and operating as a passive or aggressive dictator. The partner is reactive and submissive to the dominance of the drinker (Brown, 1988). Our questions regarding decision making confirmed this unequal and unshared process during the drinking and demonstrated how the couple moves toward greater systemic equality as a result of recovery.

The four families illustrate the process of change over time. The Corwins are in a systems vacuum: "We're not open; we don't share, and we never did." The Turners at 16 months of sobriety can talk but can't negotiate. They do not know how to differ or to compromise without fighting. As Maggie said, "We can't make it up from nothing. We don't know how to do this." At 5 years of abstinence, Roger Henderson told us, "Before, I did it my way. She could comment or not. Now we express our opinions and differences." And, at 13 years of sobriety Randy Warner said, "We don't make a decision without talking it over. We share delegating too."

The couples with longer sobriety did not just learn how to talk and negotiate. They also had the experience of healthy individual development and autonomy from which they approached each other. The emotional separation of Transition and Early Recovery pays off later.

In the early months and years of abstinence couples typically cannot tackle problems, disagreements, or feelings head-on without ending up polarized in a battle over who is right and who is wrong— in essence, who is to blame. Or one partner (in drinking, often the nonalcoholic, if there is one; in recovery, the alcoholic) gets tired of taking all the blame, as Hal Turner did. The early focus on individual growth and responsibility prepares the partners to come back later as equals and to negotiate without becoming polarized against each other.

Boundaries. A boundary is "something that indicates or fixes a limit" (*Webster's*, 1961/1981); it protects and maintains the family's individuality and autonomy. Boundaries may be fluid and loose, sometimes even almost nonexistent, or rigid and impermeable. Semipermeable (i.e., "somewhere in the middle") boundaries are the most functional, as they allow family members and others to enter or exit the system much like a gate.

In one of our families, Mom set a boundary: there would be no alcohol and no drinking in the home. Dad, who was a periodic binge drinker, maintained this boundary, leaving the home when he began to drink and not returning till he stopped. The house stayed "dry," with a safe, stable, and consistent environment for the parents and their three children. Father's drinking was acknowledged and kept separate from family life. There was a "dry" system and a "wet," drinking system (Steinglass et al., 1987), but no alcohol in the home environment.

If a boundary is too fluid, the family system is blurred, which is also called "enmeshed." Roles and rules are crossed, which may lead to chaos, confusion, and poor family function. The Warner family all described their lives during the drinking as chaotic, unpredictable, and out of control. Too rigid boundaries can result in constriction and overreliance on rules and conformity. Sometimes drinking parents exercise punitive and extreme rules with children, demanding that they demonstrate the control that the parents themselves are lacking.

Process

Process refers to communication and interactional patterns that are part of the family system (Watzlawick et al., 1974; Ackerman, Papp, & Prosky, 1970; Ackerman, 1958). Family members often want to start their treatment and recovery with a focus on communication, bypassing changes in structure. Unfortunately, their efforts to improve their communication are set within the old drinking structure that reinforced pathology. Many couples fail repeatedly because they want to avoid the collapse of the structure and the resulting vacuum that characterizes new abstinence. Yet, paradoxically, they cannot improve their communication until the structure changes.

Communication. Communication is the exchange of information between family members, which can be either effective for healthy family function or ineffective; either clear or unclear; either direct or indirect (Jacob, 1987; Watzlawick et al., 1974). Good communication leads to mutual understanding between the sender and the receiver. Ironically, clear communication itself doesn't necessarily mean "healthy" communication. Many families note that their communication was clear during drinking (i.e., it was understood that no one was to talk about drinking or any of the realities related to drinking). So, healthy communication also includes the exchange of information that maintains honesty, openness, and the fluidity of growth processes within the system, all of which is not simple. Messages must be sent in a clear, direct, and complete manner, and they must be received in a receptive and open fashion with little distortion. Communication is a two-way process, so the potential for misunderstanding and distortion of the message is always present.

We see that communication between the Corwins is very limited, not because family members are too busy focusing on their own recoveries, which is good, but because Lisa and Josh are both angry and resistant to being engaged in recovery. With 16 months, Maggie and Hal can talk more, but they need an outside professional to help them negotiate differences or facilitate a dialogue between them. At 5 years of abstinence, the Hendersons can speak openly with each other about themselves and they can positively express anger and sexuality. And, as we've seen, at 13 years of sobriety, Randy and Kay Warner talk everything over first.

Interactional Patterns. Interactional patterns refer to the dynamics of family members (Ackerman, 1958, 1994). Think of these dynamics as a dance. How do individuals move together? Is there closeness or distance, stiffness or warmth? In the Turners' first year of abstinence, Hal led the dance, which often required solo steps. Maggie wanted them to dance together rather than each alone.

Families establish their own unique patterns, which may or may not carry over to the world outside the home. For example, yelling at someone at close range may be acceptable in a family. Outside, a raised voice combined with proximity may signal a threat and a challenge. Many adults in recovery and adult children of alcoholics struggle with an internal conflict about what is normal behavior, thinking, and affect. Nothing experienced and learned inside the family seems to fit outside. The norms of the active drinking family are often defensive and extreme, leaning toward impulsive, out-of-control expression, or inward withdrawal with accompanying depression and psychosomatic symptoms. Because neither extreme translates effectively outside the home, family members must develop additional defenses to cope with the dissonance of recognizing family deviance. They may also replicate family patterns and identifications, repeating out-of-control behavior with or without any awareness of deviance. An adult daughter told us:

"I feel so awkward and even frightened in social settings. I am sure that what feels spontaneous and normal to me will be out of control, crass, and totally inappropriate."

She illustrates the internalization of, and identification with, her family's internal state of chaos and impulsive, out-of-control behaviors. She also illustrates the absence of healthy modeling.

In talking with the Warner family, we were struck by the contrast in their descriptions of chaos during the drinking years and their calm, reflective, and respectful interactions during the interview. This family was no longer dominated by impulse. They had moved from impulsive behavioral and affective expression of attachment, to thinking, dialogue, and sharing of feelings (rather than acting them out) as the cornerstones of their close relationship. This higher level of development was possible because of the autonomous growth of the individuals within the family. In the interview, no one interrupted and there was a sense that everyone was entitled to his or her own experience, perceptions, and opinions, which each expressed in turn. There was also room for healthy spontaneity.

Members of another family, with a few months of recovery, described their current experience of chaos at home. It sounded very difficult. Yet they each offered an opinion, and together weighed the pros and cons of where to have lunch after the interview, demonstrating the ability to communicate and the safety to do so, even though their primary experience was still one of chaos rather than calm.

The therapist should be alert to these positive exchanges. Noting them can be supportive to families who may feel lost in the chaos. Many newly abstinent families retain or find a healthy ability to discuss family matters and solve problems that do not touch issues of drinking, recovery, or other sensitive subjects. Dealing concretely with schedules can be immediately reassuring to family when nothing else makes sense and nothing is certain. Of course, even schedules might be out of control. The therapist looks for windows of opportunity: what kinds of things can the family address that will give its members a sense of greater safety, stability, and mastery even in the first days and weeks of abstinence. Going to meetings, making calls, and shifting one's focus to recovery provide these positive experiences for individuals.

Stability

The healthy family is able to remain stable even in the face of disruptive forces or events. The structure holds and permits the family to address, through healthy process, whatever comes along, without losing its balance, roles, rules, and boundaries (Gurman & Kniskern, 1981).

In early abstinence there is no stability at all, which is one reason why the early weeks and months feel tenuous and anxiety provoking for so many. There is no stability because there is no new recovery structure to hold the family. If all has gone well, parents have reached *outside* the family for help. It is this external support that provides temporary structure and stability while individuals are establishing the new foundation of individual abstinence and recovery. Maggie Turner collapsed emotionally and the couple relationship worked itself into a crisis when the external supports of treatment ended at 1 year of sobriety and she had no individual program to maintain her. "When the supports ended, I felt lost and became very depressed." The Hendersons, with 5 years of abstinence, and the Warners with 13 years, illustrate the internal stability achieved by families who build a new foundation and family structure in recovery.

The therapist assesses stability internally and externally, looking for strengths and weaknesses. The therapist can explain to the family that growth is a process of "fits and starts." Radical change and new learning in recovery disrupt the family temporarily. The family then stabilizes as it consolidates the new changes in behavior and identity (Steinglass et al., 1987).

Family Systems Change

A family system that is flexible can allow growth, which is a necessary part of family development. This "normal" change may take place as the family moves and accommodates itself toward a new stage in its life cycle, such as the birth of a child or when the family is jolted by a crisis. In a family with long-term recovery, clearer communication, healthier roles and rules, and a greater range of expressed thoughts and feelings are the result of individual growth and evolutionary system changes.

Most families resist change because the loss of balance and the adaptations that accompany change may be difficult and anxiety provoking. The drinking family and the family in Transition or Early Recovery resist change mightily because the unknown is so frightening: anything and everything could go wrong, especially relapse. Families do not want to be thrown "off balance" even if being stable—in balance—is very unhealthy. Many families, just like individuals, have to "hit bottom" before giving up the fight against change. It is important for families in recovery to understand that being afraid of change is normal. That's why people need so much support, and that's why sharing information and experience with others is so valuable. Not knowing where you are or what's ahead can be unbearable when you're all alone.

The therapist, as educator and coach, can provide information and reassurance. The therapist can also help the family adapt to the changes without pushing them to behave, think or feel ahead of their ability to do so. Too much pressure can activate regression and defenses, including relapse.

If changes threaten the family's stability, any member may revert to old ways in order to maintain the status quo, which may in turn literally propel the system back into the old drinking dynamics. Kay Warner told us how Sonia refused to be pulled back into a drinking family—she was sober, so she declined to drive her mother when she was drinking. In the early stages of recovery, it doesn't take much to upset the precarious new balance that supports abstinence, which is why family members are so careful not to stir the pot!

INDIVIDUAL DEVELOPMENT

According to developmental theorists, the normal life cycle for the individual is a building process that occurs along multiple lines: physiological, behavioral, emotional, cognitive, and intellectual. Despite this knowledge of multiple interactive lines of development, most mental health theories of psychopathology are limited to one track. This narrow perspective breeds controversy as professionals advocate a singular behavioral, cognitive, or affective–psychodynamic focus in theory and treatment. As we noted in Chapter 1, the goal of finding a singular explanatory theory that will provide "all the answers" has overshadowed the need to embrace greater complexity, which includes all levels and their interactions (Brown, 1985).

The narrow focus has also elevated the stature of the individual as a singular entity, separate from the developmental influence of others. Yet, a central feature of all individual development is relationship with others, particularly key figures of attachment—mother, father, and other family members. Who the individual is and becomes is a product of natural endowment (genetics, temperament, biology), individual lines of development, and the psychological–emotional bonds with family. These develop within the particular attachment, environment, and structure of the family system. Following Brown's theory (1985, 1991a, 1991b, 1991c), we emphasize the importance of all the interacting individual developmental lines, along with the interactive influence of the environment and the system.

Brown (1988, 1991a, 1991b, 1991c) advocates attachment and object relational psychodynamic theories (Bowlby, 1980, 1988; Stern, 1985; Ogden, 1986, 1989; Guntrip, 1968; Winnicott, 1953, 1960; Sullivan, 1953) as the organizing constructs that most fully address the individual intrapsychically and interpersonally. The constructivist (Guidano & Liotti, 1983; Mahoney, 1985, 1988), developmental psychopathology (Rolf, Masten, Cicchetti, Nuechterlein, & Weintraub, 1990), and trauma theories (van der Kolk, 1987; van der Kolk et al., 1996; Herman, 1992; Eth & Pynoos, 1985; Khan, 1963) also consider the interactive lines of behavioral, cognitive, and affective development for the individual, as well as environmental, interpersonal, and systemic factors.

In the developmental model, individual pathology is related to the dominant organizing influence of alcohol and alcoholism. Pathology is understood as a response—often an adaptive response—to the trauma, the system, and the disturbed attachment to alcoholic or coalcoholic figures (Rutter, 1966; Sameroff & Seifer, 1983; Sameroff, Seifer, & Zax, 1985; Greenspan, 1979; Thurman, 1985). The process of recovery is a fundamental correction, organizing new development in all three domains (see Figure 5.1, pp. 98–99). Pathology may also reflect other intrapsychic and interpersonal problems, past trauma, unresolved conflicts, and compromise formations.

Psychoanalytic theories of alcoholism (see, e.g., Wurmser, 1978; Hartocollis, 1968; Hartocollis & Hartocollis, 1980; Khantzian, 1981; Khantzian, Halliday, & McAuliffe, 1990) emphasize ego impairments and deficits, problems in affect tolerance and regression, and the use of primitive defense mechanisms. Levin (1987) advocates the view of self psychology: that alcoholism is a regression to or fixation at pathological narcissism.

In our families we see the devastating impact of parental alcoholism on children. Cary and Ken Corwin describe the trauma of living with alcoholism and their deep need for their parents to maintain recovery. Hal Turner recalls being pushed toward the "bottom" when his daughter refused to talk with him. Patsy Henderson acknowledges her neglect of her children, and Kay and Randy Warner describe themselves as absent and inattentive with their children. Many of our adults, both the alcoholic parent and the nonalcoholic, were themselves ACOAs.

There is no question that parental alcoholism adversely affects children. But it is also damaging to the adults, who adapt themselves to what they have created: a traumatic environment, disturbed family patterns, and the loss of their own growth and well-being in order to deny and preserve the drinking. All four families have told us how they did this and how they began and progressed through a recovery process by focusing on themselves as individuals.

Throughout this book, we will track the process of growth and change within each domain for the individual, the couple and family, and the children. The process of development within these domains proceeds in stages, which we turn to next.

FIGURE 5.1. A developmental model of recovery for the family.

	Drinking	Transition		Abstinence	Early Recovery	Ongoing Recovery
		Drinking	Transition			
Environment	Chronic, acute trauma; tension, anxiety, chaos, inconsistency, unpredictability, hostility; pervasive shame, guilt, emphasis on control	Intensification of chronic and acute trauma; danger		Chronic and acute trauma; chaos, crisis dominated; beginning "trauma of recovery"	Moving toward stability; still can be chaotic; hope, mixed with tension, anxiety; continuing "trauma of recovery"	Stable, predictable, consistent; not organized and dominated by crisis or trauma; supports abstinence; comfortable, secure
	Unsafe	Unsafe		Unsafe	Moving from unsafe to safe	Safe
System	Alcohol is the central organizing principle governing pathological and pathogenic family homeostasis; the family is dominated by defensive accommodations to pathology; tight, rigid boundaries; polarized relations; adaptation	In state of collapse; hitting bottom; tightening of defense; rigidity; brittle, dangerous		Collapse of system; vacuum; "trauma of recovery"; shift to external focus and support	Recovery organizes the system (Type I); split organization (Type II); no recovery organization (Type III); emphasis on separation continues; parallel lives focused on external support and attachment; foundation of new system underway	Stable, healthy new system; organized by recovery principles (Type I); capacity for self and system focus, "I" and "we," without sacrifice of either; possible family story
		Unhealthy		Unhealthy		Stable, split organization (Type II);

	produces pathology; normal tasks of family development arrested; emphasis on short-term stability in which pathology is normalized Unhealthy		Stable healthy or moving toward health		capacity for couple focus, but not organized around recovery; healthy or not healthy Stable, dry (Type III); no systems change; likely unhealthy
Individual Development	Attachment based on maintaining pathological, pathogenic beliefs, behavior, and affect to maintain system; sacrifice of individual development to systems preservation	Sacrificed to preserve endangered system; dominated by trauma; defenses against surrender; cracks in denial; despair; defeat	Shift to individual focus, which has priority over system; shift to external help, attachment to recovery; time of intense dependency; feelings of depression, anxiety, abandonment, confusion, fear, dominance of impulse	Focus on alcohol; recovery; intense education; less dominated by impulse; still new identity; still confusion; perhaps depression, anxiety; intense self-examination, self-development	Stable individual recovery; behavior, identity secure; capacity for interpersonal focus, combine "I" and "we" Spiritual development; shift from external control to internal (Higher Power); intensive self-examination, development through 12-step program, therapy, religion

CHAPTER SIX

Stages of Recovery

DRINKING, TRANSITION, EARLY RECOVERY, AND ONGOING RECOVERY

THE STAGES OF RECOVERY FOR THE FAMILY: AN OVERVIEW*

The family follows similar stages to the individual in recovery, but there is greater complexity. We will summarize the stages now, outlining the major focus for family members within each domain. This section will serve as an introduction and overview to the detailed descriptions of the stages given in Chapters 8–11 (Part IV).

None of the identified alcoholics in our research were drinking when we interviewed them because our study was about abstinence and recovery. Yet we include a complete review of the drinking stage to provide context and contrast for all the change that follows in recovery. Our families told us "what it was like" when they were drinking, so we had a "before" and "after" picture. That was the only way we could ascertain and document that any process of change had actually occurred.

Although we know that many readers are familiar with the

---

*This summary is adapted from Brown and Lewis (1995). Copyright 1995 by Jossey-Bass Inc., Publishers. Adapted by permission.

pathological and pathogenic dynamics of drinking, we will include a detailed review of active alcoholism throughout the text because drinking and all the realities of the drinking past become the key organizers of the developmental process of recovery. Families in a recovery process (i.e., a process of in-depth change and growth) can make the past real (Brown, 1991a, 1991b, 1991c); they are able to talk about drinking and do. Families in 12-step programs and/or therapy, incorporate the realities of the past into a narrative, the "story" of what happened when one (or both) adult(s) was (were) drinking or involved in the pathological drinking system. The story becomes the foundation for new development based on incorporating the realities of the past with changes in behavior and beliefs in the present. Recovery is not a developmental process separate from drinking so that the drinking past can simply be ignored, or split off from memory and experience. This way of thinking creates new pathology in which the past must be obliterated. A wish to exclude the drinking takes away a sense of foundation and an ability to see and register reality. It can lead to confusion, denial, depression, and a sense of being ungrounded in recovery. Many therapists and their patients approach abstinence from this view, however. They want to bypass drinking, to put it aside, and even forget about it, often in the service of paying attention to improving communication and all aspects of family relationship. As patients often say, "I'm not drinking, so why do I have to think about it. I want to accent the positive."

Importantly, most change in these families has not been abrupt, except perhaps for the sudden end of drinking. Yet, even abstinence is preceded by "getting ready" for abstinence—the road to "hitting bottom" that involves the end of drinking and the move to abstinence. The drinking and the "getting ready" for sobriety become the core of the recovery story: much of recovery is reversal *and* new development on a foundation of abstinence and the acceptance of loss of control. Including drinking reinforces this reality and its permanence as the organizer of recovery.

Change is a process. So, even though none of our families were actively drinking, they demonstrated how "drinking" environments, "drinking" family systems, and "drinking" individual dynamics continue into recovery as part of the normal incremental process of change. With her husband sober for 10 years, one woman remarked that it had been a long, slow process:

"I still have problems with trust. It comes in clumps. I was so burned in drinking and early recovery by the lies—I'd catch him. It felt like layers of him coming through like hidden sleaze. I went from naive to wary early on."

People in AA refer to the "dry drunk," or "stinking thinking," the return of aspects of the active alcoholic experience, minus the behavior of drinking. Many of our research families showed us the same thing: how they continue to foster drinking environments and systems, which is normal to the evolutionary process of change but which can also slow or arrest the momentum of growth. We noted in Part I how difficult it is for the family and the therapist to know what is normal to recovery and what is a problem to be addressed.

For example, Hal and Maggie Turner lived with tension, anger, and the potential for a physically and emotionally explosive encounter for 16 months of abstinence. They brought unresolved individual issues from the past to their couple relationship during the drinking and in recovery.

The Corwins still live with an arrested environment and family, system and with unchanged individuals; no recovery movement is underway. They are the equivalent of the individual "dry drunk" (Alcoholics Anonymous, 1952, 1955; Brown, 1985): no one is drinking, but all domains are functioning with drinking dynamics.

Another couple had been moving in recovery at the environmental level, which became physically and emotionally safer, over several years. Yet this couple arrested the process of change at the systems level when they decided, at 8 months of abstinence, to stop going to AA and Al-Anon meetings and to rely on each other for support instead. As the system returned to its dominant focus, autonomous individual development that might threaten the couple bond was sacrificed.

Some family members begin recovery while others lag behind or resist, creating a family environment and system that are organized by opposing realities: part of the family acknowledges alcoholism and is moving in a process of recovery organized by this new belief; other members remain organized by the belief that alcoholism does not exist. People in this kind of family are often in perpetual conflict.

Although Maggie Turner did not deny that Hal was alcoholic, she continued to view Hal and his alcoholism as the organizer of her self and her life experience. He wanted her to identify as a separate contributing participant in their couple relationship, which Maggie began to do after what both referred to as Hal's "explosion."

Let's move now to the stages. We'll continue to refer to our four families as we summarize the four stages.

STAGE 1: DRINKING

In the Drinking stage, the family is caught in the double bind of active alcoholism. They are dominated and organized by the realities of drinking, which everyone must deny and explain at the same time. In essence, the family says, "There is no alcoholism, and here is why we have to drink ... because of the stress of Dad's job, because the children fight, or because Mom is such a rotten wife."

The family focus is defensive:

- To maintain denial of any problem with alcohol
- To maintain a core belief that there is no alcoholism and no loss of control over drinking
- To invent explanations for the alcoholic reality
- To cover up and maintain the family secret

The task of therapy during drinking is to challenge defense:

- To develop and work within a therapeutic alliance that sup-ports challenging denial and acknowledging the realities of alcoholism
- To focus on the behaviors of drinking and the distorted, defensive beliefs that maintain it

The therapist may use a historic, psychodynamic frame to help family members understand the meaning of alcohol, the meaning of recovery, and their resistances to moving to abstinence and recovery. The therapist helps family members recognize their attachment to alcohol and/or the alcoholic and the dynamics of the drinking system that maintain the pathology of drinking.

The primary focus in the Drinking stage is on alcohol and the drinking behavior. The alcoholic has lost the ability and perhaps the desire to stop drinking, and the coalcoholic family members cannot control the alcoholic. Core beliefs are (1) there is no alcoholism and (2) there is no loss of control of drinking.

All four of our families described their drinking and their efforts to deny or minimize it. The Corwins included drinking as part of their regular social life. Lisa told us, "I thought we had a normal suburban life. We drank, but so did everyone. We went to work and had a good life . . . lots of friends, lots of partying, and it all seemed normal to me."

Lisa and Josh maintained denial of loss of control, believing instead that Josh had a psychiatric illness that would explain his behavior.

The Corwins described their long process of breaking denial as the individuals in the family moved toward "hitting bottom," the point at which they could go no further "down" and finally saw the truth. At the end of the road, Lisa challenged Josh: "I called in the family. We told Josh that he had to go to treatment for alcoholism or I would leave."

Why do people have to go to "the end"? Partly, at least, because people unconsciously fear that the truth will be cataclysmic. To acknowledge the truth will mean the end of this family system, which was formed, or at least adapted, to maintain denial and the pathology of drinking. People are correct in sensing the threat to the status quo of their couple and family systems. People also fear that their relationships will end, which is not necessarily true. Yet, at this point in their development, the sense of self, relationship, and the system are often the same. What is threatening is individual separation from the pathological drinking system, as well as the development of an autonomous sense of self outside that system.

Maggie Turner described her downward course: "I can see that alcoholism was always there. . . . I was hyperalert for the sounds of drinking . . . the refrigerator door opening, ice. I wondered if we'd be able to have conversations or if he'd be too drunk. . . . I'd get up in the night to see if he was alive."

Hal Turner said: "Everything progressed. I was physically addicted to alcohol and very depressed."

Kay Warner described the pain of being alcoholic: "There was a lot of insanity. I wanted to escape emotionally so I would not feel or care. I was a binge drinker, so I never knew where it would take me. I drank to the point I didn't think about anything. I would lose time and be in a blackout all the time . . . the atmosphere was insane but I had no idea." As we know, the family lived with two realities— several sober members and several drinking—for years into the recovery process.

Working with many drinking families presents a tremendous bind for the therapist: the family seeks help for another problem they wish to solve. At a conscious level, they do not want to look at alcoholism or challenge their defenses. Yet the therapist must recognize the drinking and work to highlight it as pathology—in fact, the central problem. The therapist allies with the unconscious desire of the family to get better (Weiss, Sampson, & the Mount Zion Psychotherapy Research Group, 1986; Weiss, 1993) before they can recognize the problem. In some families, the drinking is identified but the family hopes the problems of drinking will go away or get better with help.

The therapist usually does not see people and families in treatment unless some problem has been identified. It may be a problem with the kids (e.g., behavior difficulties or school issues) marital distress, or anxiety and depression that brings a family to therapy. It is the therapist's job to recognize the alcoholism and challenge the family's defenses against seeing it. The therapist should anticipate a worsening of family stress and problems as the therapy proceeds and the family moves into Transition. The therapist should also expect the environment to become more chaotic and the system more stressed and rigid as family members try to hold it together. Individuals will experience greater anxiety and more identified problems. These are a real response to the weakening alcoholic system, and they may also serve to divert attention from the alcohol. The therapist works to foster the destabilization and even the collapse of the drinking system. The therapist knows that things will not get better yet, and in fact not for some time.

The individuals or family often have come for a "quick fix" and so likely will resist the destabilization or "getting worse" that indicates a move toward Transition and "hitting bottom."

Domains

The family is dominated by an "alcoholic *environment*," an atmosphere and "context" of living characterized by anxiety, tension, and all the trauma of active drinking. The family denies the drinking and its consequences as the *system* becomes increasingly rigid and organized around alcohol. New information regarding what drinking is doing to the family cannot be acknowledged because it poses a threat to denial. Instead, the family accommodates to the drinking, altering behavior and beliefs to maintain the drinking system. For example, Lisa Corwin drank along with Josh and believed they both were "normal suburban drinkers." *Individual* growth and well-being are sacrificed to the needs of the unhealthy alcoholic system. All family members may develop what we call a "false self" or "defensive self" (Brown, 1995c), a self-view, identity, and experience organized and dominated by adaptation to alcoholism. This may become an "overlay," covering the individual's real self (i.e., the self that is separate from the dynamics of alcoholism). This overlay is what used to be called the "alcoholic personality"; for the coalcoholic partner, the overlay covers what used to be thought of as a pathological personality type—the kind of person who would tend to choose an alcoholic mate.

Adaptation to alcoholism and to being alcoholic produces defenses such as denial, projection, grandiosity, and omnipotence that are often mistaken for personality or character traits. Partners also develop defenses to cope with the reality that must be denied. For children of alcoholics, this defensive self often fuses with, or becomes, personality or character. That is because the child's "normal" development is shaped by the organizing influence of alcoholism and its defenses (Brown, 1988, 1991c, 1995a, 1995c).

In all our research families we saw the breadth and depth of trauma. By the time the alcoholic stops drinking, everyone in the family has been seriously affected and most likely become part of the system that perpetuates the trauma. On the way to abstinence, things can get very bad and usually do, with increasing stress before the denial and other defenses ultimately collapse.

The therapist assesses the organizing role of alcohol in each domain and the strength of the individual's and family's adaptation to it. The therapist assembles a portrait of defenses that maintain the pathology, a portrait that the therapist uses to determine interventions. The therapist is looking for weaknesses in the defensive structure. What is the greatest fear: that the children will be hurt; that a career will be ruined; that Mom will be arrested for drunk driving? Have any of these dreaded things now happened? What beliefs have been cherished that are being lost? What core principle in the family's self-image has been shattered? For example, the therapist hears that, in this family, being alcoholic would mean that the adults had failed to be good parents. The therapist gathers information to bear this worst fear out and presents it to the parents.

In an outpatient therapy, the therapist works to challenge the defenses in an unfolding process, careful to weigh the family's capacity to accept the reality of drinking as a problem. The family that is already in Transition and perhaps in crisis may be ready for direct challenge and perhaps entry into a structured, formal treatment.

STAGE 2: TRANSITION

The individuals and/or family are beginning to recognize the reality of alcoholism and the loss of control. That is, the alcoholic cannot control his or her drinking and the coalcoholic cannot control the drinker. The individuals or family may begin to challenge the old beliefs and behaviors that supported drinking and denial; they are moving toward "hitting bottom" and surrender, and one or more family members have become abstinent. Transition includes both the end of drinking and the beginning of abstinence.

The family focus at the end of drinking is predominantly defensive:

- To contain an increasingly out-of-control environment
- To tighten defenses to prevent or forestall systems collapse
- To maintain denial and all core beliefs that sustain it

The family focus at the beginning of abstinence is also predominantly defensive, but now in the service of maintaining abstinence:

- To focus intensely on staying dry
- To stabilize the out-of-control environment
- To allow the system to collapse and remain collapsed
- To focus on the individuals

The primary tasks of therapy are as follows:

- To break through denial
- To realize that family life is out of control
- To begin and continue a challenge of core beliefs

- To hit bottom and surrender
- To accept the reality of alcoholism and the loss of control
- To allow the alcoholic system to collapse
- To shift the focus from the system to the individuals, who begin detachment and individual recovery
- To enlist supports outside the family (e.g., AA, Al-Anon, treatment centers, therapists)
- To learn new abstinent behaviors and thinking
- To learn and practice relapse monitoring
- To explore the past and/or present, including issues of childhood trauma, utilizing psychodynamic psychotherapy if movement toward abstinence is stalled or individuals cannot maintain abstinence
- To reestablish or maintain attention to children; to maintain parenting responsibilities or ensure substitute care for children

In Transition, denial is breaking down. As it crumbles, individuals begin to feel despair. Next, they "hit bottom," which some people define as the experience of reaching the end. Sometimes "hitting bottom" is a crash that catastrophically affects everyone. Sometimes it is quiet and unobtrusive. No one but the individual knows. People who define themselves as "in recovery" describe some kind of turning point at which they knew the fight for control was over. Some also say it was the end of their fight to defend themselves against knowing reality. Although many people move into recovery at this point, some do not. Our research families told us that they were stalled until they could "surrender."

People define surrender as the emotional acceptance of the end of the battle. Surrender is accompanied by the deep acceptance of loss of control (Tiebout, 1949, 1953). Several of our families described the moment of surrender and clarity about drinking and loss of control. Hal Turner said, "I knew I was going to die so I went to the hospital." Kay Warner recalled, "One day I had a moment of clarity and I knew alcohol was my problem."

Ideally, the system will also "hit bottom," which may be why the couple seeks help. In such a system, the therapist hears that both partners feel despair: nothing works, and they accept that they cannot fix it; each has become willing, or is working toward becoming willing, to accept responsibility for change; both see themselves as "identified patients" in the sense that they recognize they need help individually;

and both accept "loss of control" and are willing to accept outside help.

The onset and beginning weeks of abstinence are a time of emotional vulnerability and dependence on external supports such as AA, Al-Anon, and a sponsor. Individuals or family as a whole may shift from drinking to nondrinking and sometimes back and forth until abstinence becomes a steadier condition. They develop new behaviors to cope with impulses to drink or to control the partner such as calling a sponsor, going to a meeting, or taking a walk. All family members are learning to disengage from old behaviors that locked them into an unhealthy drinking system. Recall how Patsy and Roger Henderson reached out to meetings and sponsors, facilitating the quick breakdown of their alcoholic couple system. They were told to stay out of each other's business, a piece of advice they could not have figured out for themselves. Because they cared about each other and were bound in an unhealthy dependence, they would more likely have wanted to be involved in helping each other. It is *very* difficult to see that the best help is for each individual to focus on the self.

Individuals in recovery begin to develop new friends and activities that are centered on abstinence and the support of a 12-step program rather than drinking. Those in recovery may feel they are abandoning old friends and family who do not fully support abstinence or who have not also embarked on their own individual recovery. This can be particularly difficult for couples in which only one partner is in a process of recovery, or the partners are out of sync, or one is further ahead than the other. The Corwins are dry, but they are not moving in a recovery process. They demonstrate so much anger with each other that they cannot shift the focus to their individual recoveries.

There can be a deep sense of loneliness and loss. Maggie Turner said, "I realized he was going down a recovery path and I'd be left behind if I didn't get a program for myself."

Some people cope with these expected, normal feelings, which are shocking and painful, by returning to alcohol. Some couples separate physically. Others weather change and the threat of change within the family, relying on the experience of people outside the family for support.

Individuals may also be struggling with new concepts of surrender and a Higher Power (Brown, 1985, 1991a, 1993). These concepts, and the idea of "spirituality," may threaten the individual still clinging to the core belief in control, or they may threaten the family that is so near to collapse as a drinking system. Surrender and the vesting of attachment and dependency in a Higher Power permit a yielding to and an acceptance of loss of control that opens the way toward positive, healthy growth in recovery. It is the vesting of dependency outside the self and outside the system that enables individuals to hold onto the experience of "hitting bottom," with its openness, vulnerability, and deep awareness of human limits—awareness of the inability to control one's drinking or the drinking of another. The belief in "something greater" than the self provides reassurance and safety. Individuals do not have to seize behavioral, cognitive, or emotional control, achieved by a return to drinking and/or a return to the belief in the power of self (Brown, 1993).

Domains

In Transition, the family remains dominated by an alcoholic *environment* that may be more stressful, frightening, and traumatic than the stable drinking period. Each of our families described how they and the environment got much worse on the way to abstinence and during the first days and weeks of being dry. The alcoholic family *system* collapses, allowing the family to shift radically from preserving the unhealthy alcoholic system to *individual* development in recovery. As we noted in Part I, there is great variability in degree of systems collapse. The Hendersons best illustrate the full collapse. For the other three families, the shift from a systems focus to individual recovery was a slower, more incremental process. Half of the Warner family was in stable, healthy recovery before Dad fully embraced recovery and the last child stopped imbibing alcohol and using other drugs.

Relapse

Relapse is most likely during Transition and Early Recovery, though it can occur at any stage (Katz & Ney, 1995; Marlatt & Gordon, 1985; Gorski, 1990; Rudy, 1980). Relapse is a return to drinking, which may also be accompanied by a drinking mind-set, a restored belief in the ability to control one's drinking. The impulse to drink becomes greater than the desire and support for abstinence. To avoid relapse, the alcoholic must have good external support (AA and a supportive environment), the ability to substitute new behaviors for drinking, and the knowledge of how to remain sober ("work the program").

Our four families illustrated how they do this by going to meetings and focusing on the new learning of recovery. We see that the Corwin family is most threatened by relapse because Josh is so newly abstinent and they are all resistant to being engaged in recovery. We expected something to happen that would move, or even shock, the Corwins into a recovery process or send them back to drinking. (We later learned that several months after the interview Josh relapsed.)

Relapse for the coalcoholic partner includes the same shift back to "drinking" behaviors and perhaps a "drinking" mind-set. A partner struggling with the individual issues in recovery and the sense of disengagement from the alcoholic that accompanies recovery may long for a return to drinking as a way to reinstate an illusion of closeness. Although Maggie Turner wanted closeness, we cannot say she relapsed in the first year because she had not yet entered recovery.

STAGE 3: EARLY RECOVERY

Early Recovery is characterized by steady abstinence, with new attitudes, behaviors, and thinking becoming integrated. The main change from Transition is a reduction in craving and impulse. Individual development continues to take precedence over the family system. The family focus is as follows:

- More congruent with the primary tasks of therapy if the family members are committed to recovery
- Fragmented, resistant, and more defensive if one partner is in recovery and the other is not, or if neither partner is in a recovery process

The primary tasks of therapy are as follows:

- To continue to learn abstinent behaviors and thinking
- To stabilize individual identities—I am an alcoholic, or I am a coalcoholic, and I have lost control
- To continue close contact with 12-step programs and begin working the steps

- To maintain a focus on individual recovery, seeking supports outside the family
- To continue detachment and a family focus guided by individual needs
- To reestablish and maintain attention to children; to maintain parenting responsibilities

New behaviors are continuously being developed and expanded to support sobriety. It is a time of action, which helps individuals cope with uncomfortable feelings and impulses to drink or return to co-alcoholic behaviors. People are advised to act quickly and automatically in favor of self-protection: reaching outside the self, usually away from close family relationships, to make a call or attend a meeting. These prorecovery actions can still be upsetting to family members who want the person's attention and may feel hurt and competitive with the 12-step, church, or therapist "outsiders" network. Yet only when new behaviors are solid and internalized can recovering individuals move from action to reflection, insight, and inner exploration through working the 12 steps.

Early recovery is a period of emerging emotions that may feel out of control. Patsy Henderson said, "I was nuts for 2 years and still not good at 3 years. I felt chaos and was always asking myself, 'Can I take one more thing?' " Individuals cope with emotions through the structure of the 12-step programs, learning to identify and name feelings and accept an emotion without having to act on it or change it. The individual's new belief structure—"I am an alcoholic and I cannot control my drinking," or "I am a coalcoholic and I cannot control the alcoholic"—is more firmly in place, which also structures and contains affect. Hal Turner felt that he pushed on his emotions too soon, not heeding his wife's wish to slow down. So when Hal expressed his anger, it ended in a raging eruption.

A fear of drinking is common in Early Recovery. Initially, this fear is helpful in providing the motivation and energy to establish supports and to learn new behaviors. It also keeps the focus on alcohol, which is necessary to create a safe, sober environment. Although the Corwins had 5 months of abstinence, they were not in Early Recovery, which is why Cary felt so fearful that her father might drink again. She seemed to recognize that a recovery process was not underway for him. Josh said he didn't like all the focus on him or on his being alcoholic. This family communicated chronic tension and a threat of relapse.

Later in Early Recovery, when abstinence is strong, fear of drinking might function as a danger signal that new awareness, conflicts, or memories of the past ("more shall be revealed") are emerging. For example, "I've been sober for a year, and I'm afraid I will sabotage my sobriety now like my father, who couldn't stay sober past a year," or, as Maggie Turner put it, "I was afraid my marriage wouldn't survive all the growth in recovery."

A fear of returning to a drinking mind-set and behaviors is also common to partners. They must exercise the same attention to establishing supports and learning new behavior as the alcoholic does. Yet, if their sense of self is vested in the other—controlling or taking care of the drinker—Early Recovery may be a time of intense loss, grief, and resistance to establishing a separate identity and separate program. Many partners told us that they believed they had no problems at all and thus had no need for help. They might be glad that the alcoholic got help and, at the same time, depressed at the vacuum they felt within themselves at the loss of the drinking bond. Maggie Turner was caught in a double bind: she was upset that she had lost Hal to AA, and afraid that she would lose him forever if she didn't accept the emotional separation and begin to focus on herself. It was not possible to have the kind of couple bond she wanted; indeed, it was not possible to have a couple focus at all except insofar as Maggie and Hal could join together to support each other in their individual recoveries.

Domains

The family *environment* is becoming more stable and predictable, though some tension continues. The biggest change is still the absence of alcohol, and some members may be feeling hopeful. Neither the Corwins nor the Turners have a stable recovery environment. The Hendersons and Warners illustrate the dramatic changes in the home experience of safety, consistency, and reliability, guided by now-stable recovery values, beliefs, and behaviors.

The family *system* remains collapsed, with reliance on external supports. Attention to couple and family issues may be positive if the primary focus remains on the individuals. This is critical: some partners may be lured away from the primary focus on individual development by a premature emphasis on couple intimacy.

Basic family responsibilities, especially parenting, must be attended to. But paying attention to parenting while tabling couple intimacy can be very difficult. Parenting issues may raise past conflicts, which trigger intense involvement, which in turn spirals the couple back into old hostile dynamics. Working together, even as parents, may require outside help for a long time.

Individual recoveries are well underway, with detachment strengthened and supported by separate recovery programs. Some individuals can begin to explore healthy communication and problem solving within the couple and family. Others may need to delay any focus on the couple.

The Corwins' drinking system was maintained by unyielding hostility and anger about the past, which prevented them from focusing on themselves as individuals in recovery. The Turners' system had just collapsed at 16 months of abstinence, with Hal's rage at Maggie. They both recognized that they could not maintain the increasing tension of his being in recovery and her refusal to get a program of her own.

We know the Hendersons allowed their couple focus to collapse immediately as they both went to AA meetings and enlisted different sponsors. By early recovery they had strengthened and solidified their individual focuses enough to begin building a healthier couple system. Their involvement with their children and their shared decision making demonstrate their ability to maintain a focus as recovering individuals while being part of a couple and family. They can hold an "I" and a "we" at the same time. Patsy told us, "We didn't leave the kids alone. Others told us they'd survive, but I disagreed. They were 7, 9, and 12 years old"

All of the members of the Warner family have completed the tasks of Early Recovery, though we see that they were divided between drinking and recovery for many years.

STAGE 4: ONGOING RECOVERY

In Ongoing Recovery, individual recoveries are solid and attention can be turned back to the couple and the family. The family focus is as follows:

- More congruent with the primary tasks of therapy if the family members remain committed to recovery

- Fragmented, resistant, and more defensive if one partner is in recovery and the other is not, or if neither partner is in a recovery process

The primary tasks of therapy are as follows:

- To continue abstinent behavior
- To continue to expand alcoholic and coalcoholic identities
- To maintain individual programs of recovery; to continue to work the 12 steps and internalize the 12-step principles
- To work through the consequences of alcoholism and coalcoholism to the self and family
- To add a focus on couple and family issues
- To deepen spirituality, expressed particularly by those in 12-step programs and/or therapy
- To balance and integrate combined individual and family recoveries
- To explore and work through issues of ACOA, childhood, and adult traumas

In Ongoing Recovery, abstinent behaviors are stabilized. External behavioral controls are now internalized so that individuals can reflect on an impulse to drink or control the partner rather than immediately substituting a direct action. But people maintain recovery behaviors as well, repeating and reinforcing the "practice" of their programs. Reliance on the steps facilitates emotional and spiritual growth.

This stage is marked by developing new interests or pursuing old ones in a different and more meaningful way, developing new relationships, and expanding one's life. Some individuals construct a social life and support system that includes non-AA people, as they now feel comfortable and safe negotiating the different recovery and non-recovery environments. For others, social life remains anchored in AA and Al-Anon, particularly when both partners have strong individual 12-step programs of recovery, as is the case for the Hendersons: "We're outgoing and entertain a lot. The kids have a lot of close relationships with sober alcoholics, and they've gone to a lot of meetings."

The individual is actively developing a personal concept of and relationship to a Higher Power. This spiritual focus alters beliefs, values, and attitudes about self and others. Basic human dependence and beliefs about control are vested in a power greater than the self. This "turning over" is what people in AA and Al-Anon refer to as the spiritual foundation of their progress and maintenance of recovery. Acceptance of "loss of control" begins with drinking and soon includes, permanently, a deep acceptance of human fallibility and limits. This belief becomes the organizing structure for healthy self-development in recovery as it challenges the pathology of the belief in the ultimate power of the self. The shift in the locus of power from the self to "something greater" paradoxically moves the individual to an equal plane with others. It reduces competitive strivings and the defenses of omnipotence and grandiosity that accompany an inflated self-view. Recovering individuals now feel a more solid connection with themselves, others, and the universe (Bateson, 1971; Brown, 1985, 1993, 1995a).

Strong individual recovery lays the foundation for a return to a couple and family focus that will accent a new relationship with healthy, open communication, equality between adults, and the possibility of greater intimacy. We accent a core principle of growth in recovery: it is not possible to have a healthy couple relationship without a strong, healthy individual foundation. Much of Ongoing Recovery involves finding a balance between individual recovery and couple and family growth, as the Henderson and Warner families illustrate.

The Warners all experienced "hitting bottom" with alcohol and other drugs, or, with Randy, in his denial of Kay's drinking. In Ongoing Recovery, Kay led the way toward a second "bottom" and a second process of growth—to open up her past on a primary foundation of recovery. She sought psychotherapy to deepen and "work through" her awareness and memories as the child of an alcoholic and of having been sexually molested. Randy also faced a crisis. In making a commitment to a deeper relationship with Kay, he had to become open to a deeper relationship with himself. He too embarked on a second "layer" or process of recovery as they began couples therapy in addition to individual therapy.

Sonia and Barry told us how difficult it was to weather this second process of growth because their mother felt so bad. It was hard for them not to conclude that Kay was demonstrating "relapse behavior," or losing her "program." In many of our families with long-term sobriety, we see a paradox: building a solid program of recovery lays a foundation for deeper emotional and spiritual exploration later in recovery, which may be ushered in by crisis or emotional pain. By the time the Warners talked with us, they were past the worst of their painful process. They could report it to us from their longer-term perspective and thus see it positively.

This family underscores the importance of holding the long-term frame in understanding, interpreting, and working through short-term events and process. Equating "change" with solving problems reinforces a crisis orientation and a belief that difficulties in recovery are a sign of failure. Difficulties in recovery and, indeed, in life are normal. The short-term focus makes it very hard to accept (and use) this basic truth. It also results in failure to recognize that the slower, underlying building process and experience of being in recovery become the foundation on which further change can build.

Domains

The *environment* is now characterized by a feeling of safety, consistency, and predictability, with anxiety or tension minimal. Crises and normal living can be faced without threatening the stable environment.

Individuals can return to a focus on the family *system*, building healthy communication and more intimate relationships without sacrificing individual recoveries. Crises and normal living can be faced without a return to unhealthy alcoholic systems dynamics.

Individual recoveries are strong and growing, which sets the foundation for adding a couple and family focus (see Figure 6.1, pp. 118–122). Members of the family can maintain a strong sense of independent self while also attending to the needs of the couple or family. Ongoing Recovery permits coexisting individual development and enhanced couple and family relationships. The Warners said it all: "It's . . . like a cycle is changing with the rest of us. We're passing on recovery instead of the disease."

FIGURE 6.1. Individual assessment criteria by stage. Adapted from Brown (1985, 1988, 1995a) and Brown and Lewis (1995).

	Drinking	Transition		Early Recovery	Ongoing Recovery
		Drinking	Abstinence		
Alcoholic					
Behavioral	Loss of control; repeated efforts to regain control; dominance of impulse	Loss of control intensified	Acute, concrete focus on new abstinent behaviors and new object substitutes (e.g., going to AA meeting, using the phone instead of drinking); impulses still dominant	Less dominance of impulse; practice new behaviors of abstinence congruent with new language and beliefs Old behaviors may resurface with new addiction or threat of relapse External support continues	Abstinent behaviors secure; old behaviors may surface in relation to past or present conflict, or emergence of past trauma Abstinent action response is in place; individual responds to old behavior as an alert for rigorous self-examination External support continues, with solid internalization of behaviors
Cognitive	Dominance of cognitive defenses: denial, rationalization, projection, grandiosity, omnipotence Defensive self: organized to maintain two core beliefs: "I am not alcoholic; I can control my drinking" Defenses become an overlay, or "false self," covering the reality of loss of control	Cracks in denial, beliefs; despair, defeat; "hits bottom"; surrender; beginning of awareness of loss of control	Confirm surrender, conversion; acute, concrete focus on new beliefs, new identity, new language of recovery Challenge of old defenses in relation to drinking and threat of relapse Beginning reconstruction of past and new construction in the present: the drunkalogue or narrative	Maintain and continue to develop new beliefs and new identity as alcoholic; deepen meaning of new language of recovery; challenge defenses that threaten relapse; begin self-exploration through 12-step program and perhaps therapy Individual focus, intense education and external support	Individual identity as alcoholic secure; reconstruction and new construction continue; consistent exploration of underlying defenses, character traits, motivation through working the 12-step program, therapy, and/or religion

Affective	May be constricted or labile; control or expression of affect is sought through use of substance; affective disturbance may be a cause or consequence of drinking or may exist separately	Loss of control, other pathology intensified; increase in impulsive expression of affect against others or self Increasing depression, guilt, desperation	Contained or denied through focus on behavior and cognition; expressed through substitute behaviors, intense action focus Depression is common, or "pink cloud" elation	Beginning uncovering and expression of feelings related to drinking and past; some experience of feelings in present; depression, grief, and mourning are common prior to or as a result of working the 12-step program Affect related to past trauma may emerge; beginning self-reflective, dynamic focus	Continuing, consistent access to and expression of affect, related to past and present, including drinking and other traumas and conflicts; process is facilitated by 12-step work and perhaps intensive psychodynamic therapy Difficulties may be related to unresolved past or present issues and fear of drinking if exploration pursued
Object attachment	To alcohol	To alcohol	Shift to "external authority," usually AA; time of intense vulnerability and dependence	Object attachment, dependence vested in AA, Higher Power; begins to be internalized To books, phone, meetings; also to sponsor, principles, Higher Power Beginning capacity for intimacy with self and other	Object attachment, dependence vested in AA, Higher Power; attachment is internalized To books, phone, meetings; also to principles, sponsor, other people, therapist, Higher Power Capacity to hold sense of self and focus, with attachment to other: "I" and "we"
Coalcoholic					
Behavioral	Loss of control in efforts to control alcoholic, others; may have dominance of impulse	Loss of control intensified	Acute, concrete focus on new behaviors and new object substitutes (e.g., going to Al-Anon meeting, using the phone instead of acting on impulse); detachment from behavioral pathology of attachment to alcoholic and alcoholic system	Less dominance of impulse; practice new behaviors of abstinence congruent with new language and beliefs Old behaviors may resurface with new addiction or threat of relapse External support continues	Abstinent behaviors secure; old behaviors may surface in relation to past or present conflict, or emergence of past trauma Abstinent action response is in place; individual responds to old behavior as an alert for rigorous self-examination External support continues, with solid internalization of behavior

(cont.)

119

FIGURE 6.1. (*cont.*)

	Drinking	Transition		Early Recovery	Ongoing Recovery
		Drinking	Abstinence		
Cognitive	Dominance of cognitive defenses: denial, rationalization, projection; defensive self organized to maintain two core beliefs: "I am not coalcoholic; I can control the alcoholic" Defenses become an overlay, or "false self," covering the reality of loss of control	Cracks in denial, beliefs; despair, defeat; "hits bottom"; surrender; beginning of awareness of loss of control	Confirm surrender, conversion; acute, concrete focus on new beliefs, new identity, new language of recovery Challenge of old defenses in relation to alcoholic and alcoholic system Beginning reconstruction of past and new construction in the present: the "story" or narrative	Maintain and continue to develop new beliefs and new identity as coalcoholic; deepen meaning of new language of recovery; challenge defenses that threaten relapse; begin self-exploration through 12-step program and perhaps therapy Individual focus; intense education, and external support	Individual identity as coalcoholic secure; reconstruction and new construction continue; consistent exploration of underlying defenses, character traits, motivation through working the 12-step program, therapy, and/or religion
Affective	May be constricted or labile; denied, displaced, projected; depression, anxiety, anger, and rage	Loss of control; other pathology intensified; increase in impulsive expression of affect against others or self Increasing depression, guilt, desperation	Contained or denied through focus on behavior and cognition; expressed through substitute behaviors, intense action focus Depression, anxiety more common than "pink cloud" elation	Beginning uncovering and expression of feelings related to drinking and past; some experience of feelings in present; depression, grief, and mourning are common prior to or as a result of working the 12-step program Affect related to past trauma may emerge; beginning of self-reflective, dynamic focus	Continuing, consistent access to and expression of affect, related to past and present, including drinking and other traumas and conflicts; process is facilitated by 12-step work and perhaps intensive psychodynamic therapy Difficulties may be related to unresolved past or present issues and fear of drinking if exploration is pursued

	To the alcoholic			
Object Attachment	Shift to "external authority," often Al-Anon, family treatment, therapist, or religion; time of intense vulnerability and dependence	Object attachment, dependence vested in Al-Anon, Higher Power; begins to be internalized; To books, phone, meetings; also to sponsor, principles, Higher Power; Beginning capacity for intimacy with self and other	Object attachment, dependence vested in Al-Anon, Higher Power; attachment is internalized; To books, meetings, principles, sponsor, other people, therapist, Higher Power; Capacity to hold sense of self and focus, with attachment to other: "I" and "we"	
Children	[These criteria are approximations and possibilities. The experiences and adjustments of children are dependent on their parents' total experience and their own development. Individual assessment of each child and each family is essential.]		[In Early and Ongoing Recovery, behavioral, cognitive, affective, and object attachment criteria are all dependent on multiple, interacting variables, including the safety of the environment, the health and stability of the system, and the parents' individual recoveries and couple relationship. The following is a general summary.]	
Behavioral	Sometimes behavioral problems; acting out; drinking; use of other drugs; Psychiatric behavioral disorders	Trauma, out-of-control behavior and experience intensified	Behavioral problems may continue or begin in response to "trauma of recovery"	Depends on age, experiences of Drinking and Transition with both parents; Depends on degree parents could focus on their recoveries and pay attention to children's needs at the same time; Children's adaptation to recovery depends on stabilization of safe environment, new, healthy system and solidity of parents' recovery	Depends on age, experience of Drinking, Transition, and Early Recovery with both parents; With secure attachments to recovering parents, children can focus on themselves, repairing developmental arrests, and building healthy sense of self; Opportunity for repair of family bonds; new experience of self and others
Cognitive	Dominated by defenses of family; develop same cognitive–perceptual distortions as parents; Also cognitive disturbance because of denial of reality	Intensification of cognitive disturbance	Often confusing, frightening; depends on parents' own involvement in recovery and their explanations; Parental congruence about what is reality fosters new construction and repair		

(cont.)

FIGURE 6.1. (cont.)

| | Drinking | Transition | | Early Recovery | Ongoing Recovery |
		Drinking	Abstinence		
	Difficulty concentrating; hyperactivity; dissociation processes		Absence of parental congruence may intensify conflict, problems	Children may still feel abandoned, frightened, and confused, or they may be settling into greater trust and hope with stronger, healthy attachment and relationships to parents	
Affective	Development is adaptation to pathology of alcoholic parents, environment, and system	Feeling of impending doom, disaster; absence of physical, emotional safety	May be frightened; need for safety, structure, and reassurance	Children may need support and help with past and present traumas	
	May be expressed through behavioral disorder or childhood emotional disorder: depression, anxiety, sleep disturbance	Increased childhood disorders	May be expressed through behavioral disorder or childhood emotional disorder: depression, anxiety, sleep disturbance		
	Trauma is normalized; need for safety, structure, reassurance; high vulnerability to stress		Trauma remains chronic and normalized; high vulnerability to stress		
Object attachment	To alcoholic or coalcoholic parents and to alcoholic environment and system	To alcoholic or coalcoholic parents and to alcoholic environment and system	Remains with alcoholic or coalcoholic parents, but children may be/feel abandoned to parents' focus on their recoveries		

CHAPTER SEVEN

Factors That Influence Recovery

W hile much happens in family recovery that is predictable and similar, there is also great variability between families in concrete experience, individual history, and life circumstances. It is important for families to listen and look for what fits in the experience of others and to recognize what doesn't. The same is true for therapists. How you listen, what you listen for, and what you do with the information are critical. You must monitor expected changes within the domains and stages, and differences in pattern that affect the normal processes. In addition, there are interactions between the stages and domains. What is the impact of the environment on the system and the individuals, the system on the environment and individuals, and the individuals on the environment and system? And what is the impact of stage on all of these interactions? Clearly, there is no easy formula. For example, Transition likely brings increasing chaos to the environment, along with the collapse of the system. Individuals may become so frightened that they defensively retreat. Their reaction to the trauma of early abstinence then slows their movement. If all members of the family, or at least both adults, are in recovery, there is explicit or tacit approval for the process of change. The therapist can reassure family members that the chaos and uncertainty are normal, monitor the family's attachments to recovery, and get out of the way of the normal process. If both partners are not in recovery, there is likely to be more stress, conflict and resistance to the natural flow. The

therapist becomes more active in pointing out resistance and explaining to the family the strong differences they are experiencing. The
therapist may need to actively support one person attending a 12-step
program when other family members refuse. With knowledge about
the normal process, the therapist can strongly suggest that all family
members be involved in some form of outside support and help them
explore their resistance.

There are also important variables that will have an interactive
impact on the process of recovery. These include participation in AA
and Al-Anon, the meaning and role of the 12-step programs, a
generational history of alcoholism, and childhood and adult traumas.
The therapist must also assess for dual or multiple diagnoses. These
might include preexisting conditions or problems that have arisen in
abstinence or resulted from it, such as depression and anxiety. Thus,
it is important to take a complete psychiatric history for all individuals,
as well as a thorough history of drinking, and a traditional biopsycho-
social profile.

Since no two families will ever be alike, it's impossible to anticipate particular details about each one. Therefore, it is important to
view each family as unique: the people in this unit have a life history
that is all their own. What they share with others is the family
experience of alcoholism, as well as patterns of family relationships in
drinking and abstinence, which do have commonalities. Many individuals and families find the sharing of experience profoundly helpful
and healing. Identification with others is an important part of reducing
isolation and providing a deep sense of safety and holding. If others
have been there and survived, there is hope. This is one of the key
therapeutic factors in AA (Alcoholics Anonymous, 1955).

Yet, within families, finding commonality and agreement may be
especially hard. Questions about drinking and recovery are often
controversial. We saw that families could tear themselves apart over
differences as to who is in recovery, who is not, and who should be.
Many families maintain a hostile, warring stance from drinking into
recovery. They argued about drinking before, and they argue about
recovery now. Many intense interpersonal struggles regarding autonomy versus control are still waged around the organizing principle of
alcohol. Is drinking to be denied in this family? Will breaking denial
cause a rupture in family bonds? Is recovery to be the norm that
everyone follows? Is the alcoholic to go alone, with others resistant to
change or content with no change? Who is in charge of defining

reality? What is the truth about drinking and about everything else? Some families embrace recovery and turn themselves over to change that is organized by an alcohol recovery focus. The Hendersons are an example. Other families fight what feels to them like more control, more dominance, and a loss of self with such a strong emphasis on recovery. We saw a complete resistance to any focus on family recovery in the Corwins. In all our research families, we saw that resistance to recovery was most acute, and the battles for control of family norms and identity the strongest, when unresolved issues within the family or from the past intruded. Often, these issues were unacknowledged and could not be dealt with openly. Family violence, past and present, infidelity, childhood trauma, and the alcoholism of others in the family are examples.

The therapist watches globally: How do family members see, think, and feel about recovery? Is one domain or stage central for the whole family, or are family members focused in different domains and stages? The therapist may intervene in a predominately behavioral mode for all of the family or accent behavioral change for one member and help another identify the interference of childhood trauma. Even though the therapist may never see the entire family, he or she attempts to monitor the whole, knowing that the members' adjustments to recovery will have a major impact on the individual and vice versa.

It is unlikely that most therapists will see families through all phases of recovery. Some may work with a family or individuals within it during drinking and long enough into recovery to see the profound changes we've described. But often therapists only work with drinking patients or those who are newly sober. Although more people in Early and Ongoing Recovery are seeking psychotherapy, they and their therapists may not have enough experience with short- and long-term recovery to know what is normal and to assess what is not, or at least what needs attention. In that case, it is just as hard for the therapist to trust the evolving process of change as it is for the family to do so.

While the domains and stages provide a map for charting the natural processes of recovery, they are only a guide. Given the huge variability in the needs of individuals, variability within the family, and variability in the role and task of therapy, individualized family assessment is essential. Our matrices of the domains and stages in Chapters 5 and 6 (Figures 5.1 and 6.1) provide an outline for assessment of the process. In this chapter, we will describe additional factors that strongly influence recovery which also require careful, individualized assessment.

VARIABILITY IN MOVEMENT
BETWEEN STAGES

Families can go suddenly from active drinking into abstinence as a whole unit, like the Hendersons, or the move into recovery can be a long process of gradual change, similar to what the Warners experienced. Whether the actual step into abstinence is fast or slow, most families can trace a period of decline during the drinking that, in retrospect, they recognize was a preparation for recovery. Although the Hendersons moved quickly together into abstinence, it was their second start. Five years earlier they had a crisis and stopped drinking. The immediate trouble was halted and they "went into hiding," drinking secretly until they reached another crisis. In the 5 years since then, the Hendersons had been "getting ready."

Although the Hendersons drank together and moved to recovery together, most couples are not so closely matched in movement. More frequently, one person enters recovery alone and the family lives with a split between the old pattern (drinking) and the new one (abstinence). In this scenario, there are often two (or more) versions of reality—there is no alcoholism in this family, and there is alcoholism in this family—in an atmosphere of chronic tension as family members straddle two worlds. This split can continue indefinitely; some couples find ways to work around it, and some end their relationship.

In assessing the family and determining a "next-step" interpretation or intervention, the first level is an environmental check to ensure physical safety: are the children unattended to and in danger; does violence continue into abstinence? Next, the therapist must determine what is the pattern of movement: are the parents both in recovery and supportive, or resisting recovery and fighting? And what is the impact of this movement on the environment, the family system, and the individuals within it? Is this a safe home emotionally? Is there a threat of trauma? What is the nature of family homeostasis at this point? How has the family achieved this balance? Or, if it has not been achieved, what keeps the family from stabilizing? The therapist might determine, for example, that a child acts out when Mom stops drinking, or that one partner stops drinking and the other goes in and out of recovery.

Does this particular family harden its boundaries and identity around two opposing realities, drinking and recovering, or will the split be temporary, a transitional system that is on the way to a more unified core? It may be impossible to tell. The therapist may describe this systems split to the couple and actively suggest ways around it, particularly if the hardened oppositional system has a negative impact on the children.

In one of our research families, the Jacksons, movement was stalled. The environment remained as traumatic and chaotic over 7 years of abstinence as it had been during the drinking. The system also remained divided and driven by anger. Over many drinking years, Mom had been the identified problem, the cause of misery for everyone (they told us) because of her alcoholic dominance and control. In recovery, she remained the problem. Now, family members rallied against what they saw as her need to control them. She wanted to tell the truth about the past and the present, and she wanted an abstinent family. No one was interested in joining her, and she remained alone. She believed that her husband and several children were drinking and denying it. She remained a thorn in their side.

Although Mom had already had many years of abstinence, the family had not changed much in any stage or domain. Dominated by anger and hostility about who was going to define the family's values and beliefs, especially about alcohol, the Jacksons stabilized early on in the Transition stage. Although Mom moved in her individual recovery, gaining insight about herself through working the 12-step program and psychotherapy, the family remained in an arrested state of development, with the environment, family system, and interpersonal relationships dominated by anger and resentment. In our study, we found that many family members achieved significant emotional growth and maturity over time but continued to have serious problems interpersonally.

In many of our research families, one individual led the way into recovery and others followed over time. Sonia Warner started into recovery, followed by Kay, then Randy, Richie, and Barry. Family life for the next few years, and even as long as 10 years, consisted of additional members entering recovery. Over this extended period, the individuals, the environment, and the family system gradually changed from predominantly drinking to predominantly recovering. The underlying experience of the decade was one of constant imbalance and change, keeping the family in a (largely positive) state of disruption. Without a global, long-term view of recovery, the therapist and the Warner family might well have attended only to the manifest disruption and interpreted the family's progress as poor. Instead, the therapist heard the underlying attachment to recovery and the dominance of recovery movement, and so facilitated the continuing process.

With almost 8 years of abstinence, Rudy and Carla Long maintain an arrested, polarized system. They disagree about everything, a relationship structure that seems to serve them well. Carla says she is working hard now to recover from the problems that caused her to drink: "I work hard not to repeat what I experienced and what I was taught. I don't have to be an abusive parent or wife." She and Rudy joke that they stay separate and stay watchful so as not to repeat the past.

With 8 years of abstinence, some couples might experience this degree of polarization as a problem, a failure of recovery. For others, like the Longs, it is an important safeguard. Carla's focus on being separate helps her maintain her healthier, recovery self. As soon as she and Rudy attempt a couple focus, old patterns, beliefs, and identifications surface and the two become locked into an intense, hostile struggle for control. At some point, this couple may decide that their ongoing disagreements are more defensive than they need.

We heard evidence that the polarized couples system gave Carla the degree of separateness she needed to ward off re-creating her childhood family structure. This recovery system serves the defensive function of holding the uncertain autonomy of the adult when internal pressures of the past, particularly childhood traumas, begin to surface. Recognizing that individual psychodynamic issues are contributing to the systems arrest, the therapist is likely to strongly recommend intensive individual therapy in this case.

Another family might experience a very long Transition. The alcoholic may cycle between drinking and abstinence, with the rest of the family constantly off balance and reacting. The Corwins typify this shaky foundation. Or some family members may remain stable in their own recoveries, holding onto new behavior and beliefs, while the alcoholic swings back and forth. Kay, Randy, and Sonia Warner stayed grounded in recovery, while Barry moved in and out.

In one of our research families, the mother had three hospitalizations for treatment of alcoholism over a 3-year period. During this time, she was alternately dry and drinking. The father attended Al-Anon regularly and maintained a stable, somewhat protected environment for their children. But it was a chaotic, frightening time for everyone. The uncertainty about whether Mom was trying not to drink, about to drink, or drinking dominated and controlled the environment. The family system held firm with the father's constancy, but no one could freely focus on him- or herself. Individual well-being and development were affected by an overriding sense of impending doom. This 3-year Transition put much of the individual and family development on hold. This is an example of how trauma fills individual and family space, drawing attention to the environment and system. The family becomes dominated by defensive coping rather than growth.

In some families, recovery is organized by the Al-Anon partner. Many seek help ahead of the alcoholic and are successful in establishing a recovery culture in the home, even though the alcoholic continues to drink. Brent Morris joined Al-Anon and encouraged his adult children to do the same. Everyone in the family was in recovery by the time Mom stopped drinking.

In this family we saw the dominant culture and its norms shift from the mother's alcoholism to family recovery. While Mom and her drinking still had an impact on the environment, the family system, and the individuals within it, her behavior and beliefs no longer set the standard to which everyone else reacted. She became deviant as others successfully disengaged from her and the dominance of her drinking.

Some families get caught in a crusade to bring everyone along, a pattern we saw in several families with grown children. Parents were sober and presiding over a sober home. Attention focused now on children who were drinking and creating drinking homes of their own. Thus, across generations, there was a combination of drinking and recovering families. Again, the Warner family is a good example. Their decision to have a sober home solidified abstinence as the organizer of the environment and family system. It helped them establish new roles, rules, hierarchies, and boundaries that provided the building blocks for a healthy family.

Several of our families demonstrated the importance of a declared sober home. When both parents were in recovery, or when both parents supported abstinence and a recovery process, they established a new organizing systemic norm that made the environment safer.

Drinking became more obviously deviant as family attachments were secured around abstinence.

Many of our families in Ongoing Recovery emphasized how important it was to have a long-term time frame. They described years of instability and change, characterized by turmoil and disruption, along with great gains. Many expressed awe at how they had gotten from there to here. It was sometimes hard to see the progress amid the turbulence, yet they knew that they had come a very long way and the changes they had made were monumental. They said it was vital to take it a step at a time; it was vital to let go of trying to control the outcome. They had to give themselves up to the process. As we've already noted, this is difficult to sustain without mentors who have come before and survived, and who offer ongoing support.

Yet it is the rare individual or family that doesn't initially resist the need for outside support because it feels so frightening. Reaching outside the family implies disloyalty and the potential breakup of the family, which is exactly right. That is what will happen: the breakup of the rigid, tight systems defenses and structures that maintain pathology. The family unit may or may not survive the breakup of the drinking system and all the change that follows. The therapist antici-pates the resistance and explains repeatedly, using education about recovery, humor, and examples of others' experience, why the individ-ual focus of Transition and Early Recovery is necessary: technically, to break up a pathologically symbiotic or hostile–dependent drinking system (Bader & Pearson, 1988) and to lay the groundwork for healthy individual and couple development. In nontechnical terms, the thera-pist might tell the couple that they worked very hard to keep the family together by repeatedly trying the same solutions—to no avail. For a time, can they let go of trying to solve all these problems on their own, and particularly as a couple? Can they listen to others who have been through this process of massive change and survived it, and trust that understanding and change in the system will come? Can they possibly trust that things will be OK, even though they might not turn out the way people want? The answer to these questions will almost certainly be "No" unless couples and the therapist can work within a "next-step" frame or, in the language of AA, "a day at a time."

Although time away from drinking does not itself promote change, it is a critical factor. Time without alcohol creates a space for new development to occur within the domains. Initially, awareness and the felt experience of this space can be frightening. The impulse is to "fill it up," which is exactly what people did by drinking. The spouse often filled this space by worrying about and trying to control the drinker. Early on, in Transition and Early Recovery, everyone in the family is encouraged to fill this space with participation in 12-step group programs and involvement in recovery activities. With a base of abstinence established by all, individuals can focus on self-exploration, which is the work of Early Recovery. The Hendersons and Warners illustrate this.

Without an awareness that recovery takes time, many individuals want to interrupt this individual focus, worried that there is no couple relationship at all and frightened that there may never be one. A participant in our MAPS class expressed relief to hear that recovery is a continuous and long-term process. She noted:

> "There is a common idea that recovery should take 1 year. Looking back, I can see that I had barely begun my own change and, as a couple, we were nowhere at 1 year. I remember wondering if we were doing something wrong, since we weren't 'finished.' It's reassuring to know we don't have to 'arrive' anywhere except where our recoveries take us."

She added:

> "Knowing we're in a process gives me perspective—the difficulties seem smaller, and I can settle into being patient when I know there is a bigger picture. What is so hard now will later seem like a bump in the road."

VARIABILITY WITHIN DOMAINS

The therapist listens with the multiple tracks of the domains in mind. At any point in time, the therapist can take a recovery check in each domain, in essence mapping the territory, noting strengths and positive movement, and staying alert to problems. What are the particulars regarding the environment, family system, and individual development? Is the process moving well? Why or why not? Is there need for intervention?

The critical global questions that apply to assessment of the stage also apply to the domain: To what degree does the entire family identify as recovering? To what degree do the individual family members identify as recovering? And to what degree can the individuals and the whole family focus on and assimilate a recovery process?

Is one parent alcoholic? Both parents? Some children? All of the children? What about grandparents and extended family? Most often, there is a long list covering three or even four generations—aunts, uncles, cousins—that have a relationship to alcohol and perhaps to recovery. In all four of the sample families we presented in Chapters 3 and 4, one or both parents had grown up with an alcoholic parent, a life experience that had markedly influenced their own drinking and recovery.

Has the family achieved a quick stabilization of the environment or a slow painful easing of tension and trauma? Is the environment now facilitating and supporting forward recovery movement or interfering? It may be hard to tell. One family, with members growing steadily in individual recovery, nevertheless lived with a chaotic, chronically tense and uncertain environment for years, as parents and children struggled with serious illness, business collapse and financial hardship, and out-of-control, addicted children. It seemed to them that they would never know peace. Yet they stabilized their collapsed system with outside supports early in the recovery process. Both parents participated in treatment, attended AA and Al-Anon, and maintained a unified stance that family life would be organized around recovery principles. Eventually, the environment stabilized and all family members joined the recovery-organized system.

For many families, a chaotic, crisis-driven environment is normal. Parents grew up with this chronic intensity and establish it quite naturally in their own families. This driven state may feel paradoxically safe or even comforting: struggling to solve problems or hold the family together feels more manageable than the emotional vacuum that often comes with abstinence. People are afraid they will be bored without action and intensity, which alcohol fueled. The fear of boredom is often an expression of an underlying emptiness.

Filling this new, potentially empty space by redirecting action and involvement to 12-step programs maintains the intensity for the individuals, while taking the focus off the environment and interpersonal relationship.

Similarly, the therapist assesses the system: What is the state of change? Is it stable in collapse, unstable, moving back to drinking dynamics, or forming a new structure in recovery? Is there resistance at the systems level? If so, what is the source? Is there a need for intervention? Is the system facilitating and supporting forward recovery movement or interfering with it? As with the other domains, it may be hard to tell.

Jackie and Jeff Nelson became abstinent, but neither reached outside. There was change in the environment, which quickly became stable and safe, but the system did not budge. Both agreed that they lived in a depressed, stagnated system until they sought couples therapy several years into recovery. The therapist helped them see how focused each was on the welfare of the other and how angry they were at the failure of the partner to "get better." They then explored their unconscious need to preserve this mutual hostile dependence.

The therapist also monitors individual change and development. Is individual attachment to recovery secure and the normal process underway? If not, what are the blocks? Early on, assessing resistance to the individual focus is critical. Is it in the service of establishing recovery or interfering with it? For example, most people are terrified of the new, vulnerable state of abstinence. They can focus on how to stay sober but not on much else. This intense, singular behavioral focus, which is essential at Transition, may seem defensive later on when it's time to begin step 4: making "a searching and fearless moral inventory" of themselves (Alcoholics Anonymous, 1955, 1952).

As we've seen, some individuals cannot assume a self-focus at all. They may insist that the partner is the problem or that fixing the couple will solve everything. Others shift their focus off the drinking system onto themselves as individuals and become more defensive interpersonally, not less, which is what occurred with Jackie and Jeff. They say that nothing changed from drinking into recovery. There was emotional separation then, and there is emotional distance now. In Transition and Early Recovery, the partners and the therapist walk a fine line to determine when the defensiveness is in the service of individual growth and when exploration within a couples frame might be helpful. Part of this fine line is understanding the difference between defensiveness and detachment. Initially, the two are often fused. People cannot grasp that they can detach from participating in the faulty thinking and behavior of another while not relinquishing their attachment to that individual. Later, in Ongoing Recovery, continued defensiveness, which can now be separated from detachment, may no longer serve individual growth and should be explored in a therapy process.

VARIABILITY AND FAMILY TYPE:
A SYSTEMS VIEW

Although we found tremendous variability between families, with no single picture of a "recovering family," we also found one clear parameter that predictably differentiated families: reaching outside of the family for help and maintaining outside help for an extended period of time was the single most important factor in maintaining a process of recovery. It was also a critical factor in determining whether a family had a smooth or rough Transition and Early Recovery. We have called this outside help the "external authority." This variable wielded tremendous influence over the stage of recovery and the state of adjustment and change within the domains.

In our sample, 72% of all subjects belonged to a program of recovery, almost entirely AA or Al-Anon: 86% of the alcoholics belonged to AA, and 53% of the coalcoholics belonged to Al-Anon. We had three distinct kinds of couples (Lewis, 1997), depending on their affiliation with recovery programs: Type I, in which both partners identified as alcoholic or coalcoholic (some identified as both) in recovery; Type II, in which one partner identified as being in a program of recovery and the other did not; and Type III, in which neither partner belonged to a recovery program.

Consistently, we found that couples in which both partners identified themselves as *individuals* in recovery (Type I), usually within an AA or Al-Anon frame, had "second-order" systems change (Watzlawick et al., 1974; Lewis, 1997). As we noted in Chapter 1, second-order change involves a shift in paradigm—the individuals "hit bottom," accepting their loss of control—which facilitates the transformative move to recovery. Type I couples had the most congruity between them in their views of and progress in recovery. The Hendersons and Warners are examples.

Type I couples and families demonstrate the following characteristics (Lewis, 1997):

1. They are receptive to resources and active participation in AA, Al-Anon, and/or recovery-focused therapy.
2. Each spouse accepts an "identified patient" (IP) role.
3. Recovery is a central organizing principle in all three domains.
4. There is tolerance for the loss of the familiar and hope for change.

5. A second-order change occurs as each partner perceives the need for change in all three domains.
6. There is a shift in attachment to a Higher Power, however defined.

Couples in which one partner belonged to a 12-step program and the other did not (Type II) did not experience a second-order systems change, although one partner may have experienced this transformational shift individually. As a result of uneven dramatic change, they had more ongoing conflict about their relationship and in determining what the "proper" focus on recovery and outside help should be (as the Corwins and Turners illustrated).

Type II and Type III families exhibit the following characteristics (Lewis, 1997):

1. There is only one IP (Type II), or none (Type III).
2. The family system, whether drinking or abstinent, remains closed and organized by drinking dynamics or resistance to change.
3. The couple and family are not receptive to or active in outside supports; thus there is no systems collapse and no possibility for second-order change.
4. The family is organized around defense, not recovery.

In some of our couples, the AA or Al-Anon partner worried about outgrowing the noninvolved spouse or leaving him or her behind. Hal Turner said he would set priorities, choosing AA instead of his marriage. An AA husband with 3 years of abstinence said he had grown up since he stopped drinking and he felt now as if he were graduating from high school again. Continuing with his analogy, he said sadly that his wife was still in eighth grade. Both felt a gap between them and worried about what would happen to them as a couple.

The spouse who is not in recovery may prod the 12-step partner to reduce meetings or to shift the focus of recovery off the self and onto the couple. In several families, the 12-step partner decided to end all outside help and "work together as a couple to maintain recovery." As we've said, when the couple decides to terminate outside sources of help, particularly in Transition or Early Recovery, they are more likely to return to old problematic patterns of behavior and relating to fill the vacuum that resulted from hitting bottom and moving into recovery. While the individuals may maintain abstinence, their growth as a couple may be slowed, skewed, or halted. Nobody in the Corwin family but Josh was going to meetings. Lisa, Cary, and Ken were all stuck in their old behavior patterns. Josh was too angry at them and at being alcoholic to proceed into a healthy process of recovery for himself, without his family.

As we've noted, in several of our research families, the split between partners over 12-step program membership centered on the unstated belief of the recovering spouse that the other partner was also alcoholic but not identified and therefore was still in denial in the Drinking stage. Growth in the recovery of one spouse widened the gap between the partners. Many of these families lived with intense hostility, chronic tension, and a war about what was reality and what was not. Lisa Corwin and Maggie Turner both drank with their husbands. We sensed a lingering undercurrent within both couples as to whether the women were also alcoholic and, if so, when they would come along. Some recovering alcoholics feel resentful that they got the role of IP: why should the partner get to keep drinking and not be identified as an alcoholic too?

Finally, couples who had no outside help of any kind (Type III) demonstrated little or no recovery as individuals and no systems change. These couples exhibited the most turmoil and ongoing problems in the interview. However, paradoxically, these same couples showed the most "normal" test scores on the Minnesota Multiphasic Personality Inventory (MMPI; Butcher, Dahlstrom, Graham, Tellegen, & Kaemmer, 1989) and several measures of couple and family function. In essence, the central organizing principle for Type III family members, is defense and not recovery. They have not experienced a shift in paradigm, and they are not engaged in a new process of development, guided by a belief in loss of control. These couples and families abstain from alcohol and change nothing or very little else. The defenses that maintained the drinking continue to operate in recovery. From our interview, we knew that these families were denying many unnamed and unexplored issues, individually and as couples. Many registered high scores on the defensive scales as well. In our clinical work, we would identify these couples as being at high risk for relapse. This finding will be shocking and unwelcome for many clinicians and insurers: "normality" in outward function can be defensive; relying on short-term, strictly behavioral outcomes can lead to inaccurate conclusions. Worse, striving for "normal" appearance can retard or derail the healthy but far from placid growth process of recovery.

Consistent with our model of long-term recovery, in which the couple and family experience profound, lengthy disruption to the system as part of normal development, our Type I and II couples also demonstrated less "normal" test protocols of family function. The radical change and turmoil of recovery were reflected in the measures. In the interview, these problems were more readily identified by all and openly discussed. Thus, people had less need for defense. Many had learned to accept and tolerate problems. As one couple said, "We perceive difficulties and crises as 'part of our work.' "

Importantly, the majority of individuals, both alcoholic and coalcoholic, tested within normal limits on the MMPI (Lewis & Atzmon, 1997). This finding supports the view that alcoholism produces pathology (Vaillant, 1983). Individuals in recovery resemble the normal population much more than they do the contrasting norm group of psychiatric patients or drinking alcoholics.

Couples who have had no help at all (Type III) continue to operate from the old drinking system dynamics, which they cannot change from within. The Corwins are closest to this picture. In understanding the couples' choice not to seek help, it is often useful for the therapist to ask about their past history of attendance at AA and Al-Anon, what that experience was like, the meaning of these programs, and what it means and how it feels to seek help.

RESISTANCE TO OUTSIDE HELP

In our research and in our clinical experience, initial resistance to AA and Al-Anon is nearly universal. The therapist should expect that people will not happily accept a referral to 12-step program meetings and promptly go, embracing recovery and the help it offers. What is the source of such families' resistance? Many will say that they are "private people" and prefer to deal with their problems alone or in the shelter of therapy. Others state that AA and Al-Anon are "too religious" or that these programs are for people who have lost control of their drinking and they have not. Seeking help may activate feelings of failure or threaten loss of one's deepest defensive beliefs—there is no alcoholism in our family nor any loss of control—

the core beliefs that maintain the pathology. People know intuitively that reaching outside the system will break it up. The therapist should assess whether the resistance relates more to individual dynamics, the couple, or both.

As therapists, we automatically recommend AA and Al-Anon to all such patients. When they explain why they cannot go, noting that they are different from people who go to these organizations, we might ask what they think would happen if they did go. We might also point out, with perhaps a hint of irony, that people are not standing in line to get into AA or Al-Anon, that we have never met anyone who just couldn't wait to get into AA or Al-Anon, and it is therefore amazing how many people have nonetheless found a way to make AA and Al-Anon work for them. We might also say directly that the best way to investigate whether they have lost control or not is by attending meetings and listening to see if peoples' descriptions fit their own experience. It is important to frame suggestions as possibilities and choices. Many people fear that they will lose autonomy if they identify themselves as alcoholic or coalcoholic and belong to AA or Al-Anon. In fact, the reality is just the opposite (Brown, 1985, 1993). As therapists, we might also wonder whether one or both partners would resent the 12-step involvement of the other.

While some couples and families said they participated in the research as a way of giving back what they had been given, others acknowledged that they needed help and wanted to use the interview to assess their difficulties and help them change. Identifying the alcoholism of another was only one example. Some families wanted help in talking about the past, in naming reality and starting a family dialogue. Many wanted to raise issues in the research setting that they were too afraid to identify on their own. Some feared that bringing up past abuse, hurt, anger, and unspoken truths would cause the alcoholic to drink, even with long-term recovery. Sometimes we saw families at a time of crisis, with old or new problems surfacing for attention. Or sometimes families were unconsciously preparing for a radical shift, often part of the normal process of growth—yet they were stumped somehow, or afraid.

One of our couples, Jason and Margie Greenough, with 5 years of abstinence, volunteered to participate a few months before we could schedule their interview. A week before, Margie called to say that Jason had started to drink again. Tearfully, Margie asked us not to cancel the research meeting. When she called initially she had been worried about problems in their relationship, which she hoped they could explore in the interview.

With the Greenoughs we no longer had a couple with 5 years of uninterrupted abstinence. In fact, we no longer had a couple who fit our research criteria. But we did have a couple in which one partner was relapsing, according to our definition. What could we learn? We met with the Greenoughs and, following our research protocol, learned that they had formed their relationship around addiction—his with alcohol and hers with food—and entered recovery together as well. Both had joined 12-step programs and established recovery in all domains. However, Jason had experienced serious depression for much of his abstinence, related to unresolved issues with his alcoholic father. He told us he hated to see himself as powerless; to get over this, he needed to learn to drink. Jason knew he was still an alcoholic, but he wanted to be a "soft-core" drinker. Jason further said he had changed his definition of recovery. Although he was drinking, he did not consider himself to be in relapse. Margie did. She was distraught with the rupture to their entire recovery world. She reminded him repeatedly that he had accepted his loss of control of drinking, and he told her he had been wrong. He was taking back control so he could stop feeling so depressed. She was frantic that the bond of recovery they had forged for 5 years was gone forever. Margie was afraid their marriage would not survive with such radically different definitions and perceptions about reality related to drinking.

A few months later, Margie called and asked if they could come in to view the videotape of their interview, an option we offered to all participants. Before they viewed it, Jason said that he had experienced too many problems as a consequence of his renewed drinking and had decided to stop a few weeks earlier. However, he did not believe he had lost control. He told us he would change his behavior—he would be abstinent—but he would not change his belief in his own control. Jason hoped Margie would be satisfied, but she was worried and still felt a breach between them. As Jason watched the tape, he was shocked. He pointed out his "alcoholic thinking" and acknowledged to us how defensive he had been in the interview. Still, he was not going back to believing he was powerless. For now, Margie and Jason were stabilized in abstinence, agreeing to disagree on the beliefs they held. It was a painful status quo.

The experience of powerlessness and the collapse of the self and the system that goes with it during Transition are almost always cataclysmic. Jason and Margie experienced trouble around the same issue with 5 years of recovery. Now, they had asked for help. Margie continued in her 12-step program, both were in therapy, and they had volunteered for the research.

If only one person is identified "in recovery," the "external authority" or outside help—AA, Al-Anon, therapy, or religion—is likely to be perceived as an intruder, competitor, and threat to the old relationship status quo. Lisa and Maggie both resisted Al-Anon. Maggie felt competitive with AA: "First it was liquor, and now it was recovery. I resented his meetings every night. He had no time for me." No wonder one partner in recovery wants the other partner to join.

A woman with 4 years of recovery illustrates:

"In my first year or recovery, I focused completely on myself and my husband focused more intensely on me. He was so depressed. He liked me better drinking. I told him repeatedly that he had to get some help for himself, which he finally did. For the next several years, we lived parallel lives with a lot of support for each other. After 4 years we're both still growing. We can identify our own individual issues, feelings, and needs, and we are beginning to build a new relationship together."

ADULT CHILDREN OF ALCOHOLICS

One of the most important intervening variables was a history of having grown up with an alcoholic parent (Liftik, 1995; Brown, 1994). More than half of our sample, 50% of females and 57% of males, alcoholics and nonalcoholics, identified themselves as ACOAs. Some 60% of identified alcoholics (both men and women) in our sample had an alcoholic parent (see Appendix B, Table B.4a, for greater detail). With this family history, therapists must consider that difficulties in sobriety—at any stage—will have a complicating psychodynamic and traumatic origin or component. Several of our research couples struggled with being sober because of early childhood issues. Several felt an intense loss when they stopped drinking, because a parent had never stopped. They described an attachment bond that had long been tied to drinking. Patsy Henderson recalled the loneliness she felt in her first year of abstinence because she lost her parents. Still in an active alcoholic system themselves, they did not understand why she had stopped drinking and they could not offer their support.

Ray Malone, with 7 years of abstinence, said he had always felt a special closeness to his father when they drank together. Ray told us sadly that he didn't have a reason to drink any more after his father died. He was depressed for several years of Early Recovery, missing his father and the alcohol that symbolized their bond.

Chuck Wilson, sober for several years, also experienced depression for an extended period early in his recovery. Chuck was agitated during the interview as he outlined significant emotional problems throughout his childhood and adult life. His father had stopped drinking but remained anxious, impulsively angry, and physically abusive. Chuck said his father had "raw nerves." Chuck's childhood experience of family recovery was a continuation of trauma, as was his own recovery. We could see clear signs of posttraumatic stress disorder (PTSD) emerging for Chuck after he stopped drinking as memories of his childhood were activated. He had identified with his father and emulated him. Now, in recovery, he experienced depression related to the loss of alcohol, and to the emergence of affect related to childhood trauma. We sensed that he was also afraid he would be as abusive in recovery as his father had been.

Debbie Buchanan, sober for 2 years, described herself as "in the middle" of three generations of alcoholic women. She said her mother had always been an alcoholic, though Debbie had not recognized it until she stopped drinking herself. Now, she said her mother had a fierce drive to maintain her own version of reality and that she had always been in charge of the family history. Taken together, these facts shed light on Debbie's experience of anxiety in recovery. Debbie felt that she had betrayed her mother by acknowledging her own alcoholism and becoming abstinent. Debbie's daughter, Gina, in her mid-20s and struggling with her own drinking, said that her grandmother doesn't want anyone to be an alcoholic. We could see that attachment and feelings of closeness for three generations of women had been symbolized by alcohol and shared drinking.

Here the therapist ought to note the generational history and the significant psychodynamic issues alluded to by both mother and daughter. In a recovery check, or a clinical setting, the therapist might recommend individual therapy for both to explore issues related to being an ACOA. These might include attachment, identification, feelings of guilt and betrayal about one's own recovery, and the traumatic childhood experience of parental alcoholism (Brown, 1988, 1991a, 1991b, 1991c, 1994, 1995c; Brown et al., 1989; Cermak, 1986; Vanicelli, 1989; Wood, 1987). And much more. We know that the experience of having an alcoholic parent or parents and living with parental alcoholism can be a dominant shaping influence in a child's development.

We had several young couples in which one or both partners had acknowledged their alcoholism by their mid-20s and, in their abstinence, were struggling with the trauma of alcoholic parents. While many of our research participants were ACOAs, these young people experienced their own severe alcoholism early on and had reached recovery early on as well. In a few cases, it was difficult for them to identify themselves as alcoholics and very difficult to undertake a program of recovery separate from their partners. Several of these young people credited their recoveries to spouses who had not lived with alcoholism and thus were viewed as stronger. The young couple bond was formed with the nonalcoholic partner as the protector and model, in our view making separation and the development of individual recovery programs more difficult.

The therapist in such cases would recognize the benefit for both to enter 12-step recovery programs and would cautiously recommend that, explaining why; however, these couples will most likely continue to resist the separation that follows seeking help outside the couple relationship. Individual and/or couple therapy would usually be strongly recommended as well.

DUAL DIAGNOSIS

Dual diagnosis (or, as we prefer, multiple diagnoses) is a difficult, controversial concept. While there is general agreement that people can suffer coexisting disorders (Nace, 1995; Kaufman, 1994), in dealing with alcoholism it is often impossible to determine what is separate and what is cause or effect. Establishing a primary diagnosis can be a chicken-or-egg problem. There is no doubt people drink to treat all kinds of emotional problems, such as depression and anxiety, but these disorders are also a direct result of drinking (Vaillant, 1983; Bean, 1981; Bean-Bayog, 1986). It is important to take a careful history of prior and subsequent disorders, and to tailor treatment to address all issues as they have an impact on recovery.

Many individuals in our research reported a history of psychiatric problems besides alcoholism. Some of these illnesses predated drinking, such as childhood trauma, and some were a consequence of the alcoholism. Several men had severe PTSD and depression following the Vietnam War. Others experienced depression in response to the loss of alcohol and in the loss of attachments that had been symbolized by alcohol.

A significant percentage of our sample (57%) had a history of psychotherapy prior to abstinence, and a majority (51%) had been in therapy in recovery. Our sample was highly biased in this direction, however, because many families were referred to the research by their therapists. To our surprise, we had some difficulty enlisting couples and families who did not come by way of therapists or some continuing connection to treatment programs. Although our sample numbers were small, we sensed anxiety about opening up to questions about recovery in several couples with long-term recovery who declined to participate. Several who did told us it was painful, though also worthwhile.

LANGUAGE AND THE NARRATIVE OF DRINKING AND RECOVERY

As much as alcoholism is the behavioral loss of control of drinking, it is also a thinking disorder. Individuals deny that there is any problem with drinking *and* explain it in a way that allows the drinking to be maintained (Brown, 1985, 1995a, 1995b, 1995c). The cognitive defenses of denial and rationalization maintain the pathology of drinking as a central organizing principle in the family. Language, including a particular vocabulary and structure of logic, obscures, circumvents, or rationalizes reality rather than clarifying it. No wonder families have communication problems. The denial of reality—that drinking exists and is a problem—as well as distorted thinking and explanations related to drinking all become entrenched in maintaining family members' attachments to one another and in maintaining the family's identity as a whole (Brown, 1988; Guidano & Liotti, 1983; Berger & Luckman, 1966; Goleman, 1985; van der Kolk, 1987; Krugman, 1987; Heimannsberg & Schmidt, 1993).

The use of a common recovery language and vocabulary was a significant factor in differentiating families in recovery. It was a key bridge for many couples in moving back toward a couple bond after the initial jarring separation of Transition. Several families told us they began to talk together about each of their individual recoveries using the language of the AA and Al-Anon programs. The sharing of a vocabulary organized by the experience of loss of control served as a unifying bond for couples and families at every stage. Differences in vocabulary and in ways of thinking about drinking and recovery were closely related to disagreements and divisiveness in the process of recovery. Couples whose view of reality was divided did not speak the same language anymore.

We observed the power of language to deny and shape one couple's conscious view of reality. We also heard the strain in the relationship between them reflected in their different use of language. Sally Collins had been abstinent for 8 months. When she spoke with us about herself and her individual recovery, she used AA language to describe her experience. She felt calm and clear. Listening, her husband, Ross, squirmed as he focused on the couple. He spoke about intimacy and the importance of "the relationship." Sally could not talk with Ross about her recovery because Ross wanted only to talk about "the couple." He did not have his own recovery, or an identity independent of Sally, which would have enhanced their separation, accomplished by her abstinence and individual development, while also permitting them to share ideas and feelings together. For now, Sally could not relinquish (and should not relinquish) her attention on herself, represented by the individual focus and individual language of AA. She became quite anxious as Ross pushed her to be closer to him.

With a similar couple, we saw signs that Brant might be struggling with his own drinking. He said he still liked to drink with his wife's mother, who couldn't be an alcoholic because she was never hospitalized (his wife, Hallie, had been). This statement demonstrated Brant's distorted thinking, or "accounting system" (Brown, 1985). When we asked Brant how he defined alcoholism, he said that alcoholics are people who end up in the hospital because of their drinking. That hadn't happened to him. Further, Brant noted that "alcohol promotes health and prevents heart attacks."

Hallie was clearly struggling with the confusion in meaning and reality. She described an indelible memory: sipping brandy from a bone china cup with her mother. Hallie misses spending time with her mother now because she (Hallie) is going to meetings.

We think that Hallie is in a precarious position. Will she be able to hold onto her new reality, including her sense of herself as an alcoholic, which means she is separate from her husband and mother, or will she drift back into drinking? In our meeting, she was holding on. But we could feel the blurring of personal boundaries as it seemed to us that Brant clearly missed Hallie's drinking with him.

With 7 years of recovery, Kelly and Seth McGovern recalled talking with each other about their programs during their first few years. It helped them support each other. Now, according to Kelly,

> "We could not be the people we are without guidelines, which have given us communication skills. Seth can tell me how he feels now, and I am safe enough to tell him. In the beginning we could only share our programs."

The language of recovery helps individuals build the narrative (or "drunkalogue") of their alcoholic or coalcoholic lives and their recoveries. In the context of Alcoholics Anonymous (1955) and Al-Anon (1984), individuals learn to tell "what it was like" (during drinking), "what happened" (to move the person to recovery), and "what it is like now" (that the person is abstinent). Over time, the narrative builds, as individuals break through deeper layers of denial and distortion. At first, couples focus on themselves as individuals, sharing and comparing what each is learning. Later, they can construct a history of their lives together organized by alcohol. Many of our research families told us they hoped the interview would help them learn to talk to each other more.

The language of addiction and recovery makes drinking and all that happened real. It lets family members build a new story of the past and to name reality in the present. Both are hard to do. One of our couples told us their hardest struggle in recovery was to figure out what the truth was. Both had lied for so long they could not tell the difference between reality and fantasy when they were drinking and they couldn't tell the difference now that they were sober. The distortion and outright lying were second nature.

We replayed one tape many times listening to the changes in language and tense. When Andy Goodwin described his drinking, he always used the present tense so that we could not distinguish between then and now. He described hiding his liquor, easing into rationalizations and murky language. He said he was sober and in the next sentence talked about drinking. Andy had lapsed into his "drinking self" as he identified with the narrative of his past. For us, it was a window to the defensive false self of the drinker. We could not tell what was real. Andy became perfectly clear as he talked about abstinence in recovery language. Our experience of a "split self" (is the person we are talking to drinking or not drinking?) was gone.

The construction of a shared narrative can bring the family together. Pressure to share the story and the language can also drive a family apart. We could see the insiders and outsiders, those who had "joined" recovery and those who had not, on the basis of shared language. One couple said it was like living in a bilingual family. They talked recovery, and their children gave each other knowing glances. Although they loved having sober parents, sometimes they could hardly recognize them.

Another couple, the Nolans, struggled over the absence of a narrative. Larry said he had a story of his drinking when he lived in a drinking world—a tale of his family growing up and his young adult years. Now, however, he is out of that system and he has no story to tell. Instead of making his past real through the creation of his narrative, he wants to shut it out. Larry does not want to think of himself as an alcoholic, nor does he want to incorporate the reality of his drinking into his conscious identity. He doesn't want to remember his past and claims he no longer has a problem with alcohol. Diana, his wife, sensed that he had transferred his dependence on alcohol to a dependence on her, which caused her great anxiety. As Larry walled off his awareness and conscious identification as an alcoholic, she became the "holder" of this reality. Diana felt silenced in working through her own experience, their experience together, and she worried about him. In our view, Larry blocked off awareness and integration of his childhood and young adult life because of trauma in his alcoholic family.

In another family we saw that progress in recovery was sharply arrested because no one was allowed to talk about the physical abuse that occurred routinely during drinking. This family could celebrate recovery, which they did, but they still had to go around the realities of drinking. Freedom to grow was hindered by everyone's awareness of the secret that could not be named.

As we proceed in Part IV to detailed descriptions of the stages, where you will hear the language and narratives of people in recovery, recall what Hal Turner said about the importance of his story and of his wife's being in recovery: "The story holds us and our lives. If we don't change, the story won't change either."

PART FOUR

A Developmental Model of Family Recovery

CHAPTER EIGHT

The Drinking Stage

In Part IV, we will describe the process of recovery in depth and detail. We'll move stage by stage, outlining the key tasks and themes for individuals—the alcoholic, the coalcoholic, and the children—and the couple and family. Now, we will pull together all the pieces we described earlier: the key assumptions underlying the research, our major findings, the summary of the domains and stages and the variety of factors that contribute to variability in the experience of recovery. The therapist listens with all of these factors in mind, assessing movement in each domain and stage, focus, variables, and barriers. In essence, this is "mapping out" the process, which the family can learn to do as well. Charting the multiple levels of recovery at any point in time is essential to accurate, thorough assessment.

The therapist will hear evidence of the multiple problems people face in abstinence, including a history of family alcoholism, trauma, past and present, and the importance of the narrative in working through all this trauma (Herman, 1992). He or she will again hear the voices of the families, illustrating how they have come to think about themselves, and to make sense of the past and present, which is reflected in the development of their own family stories.

Before we begin with the Drinking stage, let us acknowledge to readers that this chapter may seem rather familiar and even somewhat repetitive: you already know the drinking dynamics (the summary in Chapter 6 was enough of a refresher). As we stated earlier, we include the Drinking stage in detail because it is the foundation of recovery. It is not chopped off or unremembered. It is the core of the story of recovery, the "then" of "then and now." Knowing what it was like during drinking helps the therapist assess change following abstinence and to anticipate hurdles in recovery, particularly threats to maintaining abstinence, or core issues that may arrest recovery movement. However, we recognize that, despite our rationale, some readers may elect to skip this chapter. If so, we'll meet you at Transition (Chapter 9).

OVERVIEW

During the Drinking stage, the alcoholic, partner/spouse and family adjust to alcoholism as the central organizing principle for the family. It permeates the thoughts, feelings, perceptions, and behaviors of everyone in the family who must, at the same time, deny its existence. This double-bind leads to a range of different experiences, but most often to chaos, confusion, mistrust, loneliness, and isolation from self and others for all members.

Alcoholic drinking may develop rapidly or slowly over many years. Once the drinker begins to *need* alcohol, that individual and the family begin to adapt themselves to drinking and then to actively organize around it. The alcoholic engages in "alcoholic thinking," attributing problems to outside circumstances—"the boss" or "the spouse," for example. From the alcoholic's perspective, drinking may be seen as the solution to cope with these circumstances. The spouse follows the alcoholic's lead to keep peace and to maintain family unity and the attachment to the partner. The drinking is often not identified as the problem. Yet it is justified, rationalized, and minimized, a massive feat of distortion accomplished at great cost to all.

Rich and Molly Lawson, with 7 years and 5 months of abstinence, describe the process of organizing their lives around alcohol:

RICH: I was probably an alcoholic forever. I took the Twenty Questions [test] when I was 22, and I knew I answered too many yeses. So I amended my answers, changed them so I would not have so many signs of alcoholism. Even by then my life choices and daily schedule were designed to enable me to drink.

MOLLY: When it got bad, I felt that life was stopping, I felt out of control, but I defended him. My father was an alcoholic, so this life was all I knew. I couldn't see that it was alcohol.

Molly describes how her childhood family life was normalized around drinking. The therapist knows that it may take a long time in recovery to recognize that a parent's drinking was anything other than "normal" and that it had an adverse impact.

RICH: I always drank, but as it got worse and worse, I bargained with myself and with Molly. I got a motorcycle that I had wanted for years and decided not to drink. Then I decided not to drink and ride, then not to get drunk and ride, then not to get real drunk and ride. . . . I was in an accident that killed someone. It was awful, but after I was out of the whirlpool of drinking for a while I decided I could drink again.

Rich and Molly illustrate the centrality of alcohol in their lives and their accommodations to it. At this point, neither could stop it, so they had to explain it away or expand their standards for what was acceptable behavior as Rich illustrates. From a distance of 7 years, they can see clearly. This clarity of vision has been facilitated by and is a reflection of the construction of their stories, which, as we noted earlier, makes the drinking and the accommodations to it real. In working with a family in recovery, the therapist supports the continuing development of the narrative. What cannot be recognized and acknowledged as having existed in the past will continue to hamper family relationships and growth. What can be acknowledged as real can also be integrated, a process that frees the family members from their dominant need for defense.

In working with a drinking family, the therapist builds an alliance based on challenging the family members' beliefs about themselves, particularly those related to alcohol. The therapist makes the links that connect family problems to the realities of drinking and the organizing role of alcohol and drinking in the family. The therapist builds a portrait of family alcoholism in the environment, the drinking system, and the individuals within it, and presents it back to the family. Let's now examine the domains for the drinking family.

THE ENVIRONMENT

In the alcoholic environment, the daily experience for family members is filled with tension, strain, and often trauma. Psychiatrist Henry Krystal (1978) defines trauma as the "overwhelming of the self's preservative functions in the face of inevitable danger." He continues, "The recognition of the existence of unavoidable danger and the surrender to it mark the onset of the traumatic state" (p. 112).

Many people think of trauma as a single event or episode outside of the "normal" pattern of events and relationships within the family. This description fits what are called acute disasters, such as fire, flood, or earthquake, or a single episode of rape. In abusive and/or alcoholic families, the trauma is frequently chronic: a state of unpredictability, terror, and abuse is the norm. Episodes of acute trauma—violence, incest, arguments, and psychological and physical abandonment—may also occur within the framework of chronic trauma.

Other researchers have described the cumulative effects of living with trauma. Psychoanalyst Joseph Sandler (1967) suggested that the accumulation of potentially traumatic experiences could lead to a state of "mounting vulnerability." Today, the notion of vulnerability is central to our questions about trauma and its impact: what kinds of experiences lead to what kinds of consequences; how much of this experience will lead to that result; what experiences for which people create the greatest risk?

It's important to understand both the "normal" chronically traumatic environment, or "life context," of the alcoholic home and the acute traumatic events that can occur within this chronic context. This is where an understanding of the environment and the system's pathology becomes so important. Whether it's in the foreground or the background, or both, the context is traumatic.

Krystal (1978) and van der Kolk (1987; also van der Kolk et al., 1996) suggest that psychological trauma may make an individual particularly vulnerable to intense emotion. The person will respond excessively and in ineffective ways, and will overrely on defenses such as repression, rationalization, and denial of the trauma. In an extreme state, the person may be able to feel only a sense of being "dead." These individuals may feel empty, experience little or no affect or sense of depth, not recognize any wants or needs, and seek continually to fill the void within. Severe trauma may result in a paralyzed, overwhelmed state; victims may be unable to move; they are withdrawn, disorganized, and lacking their former personality traits. The most common consequence is a mixture of depression and anxiety.

Chris Weber, 23, recalls his growing-up experience with his mother, sober 9 years, and father:

"She was drinking and on prescription drugs, and Dad was yelling a lot. I was 10 and hadn't been worried before. But I knew he had reason to be upset with her; I just didn't know why. I was scared and stayed away if I could. At times I was more upset with his anger than her drinking. I didn't get loving care, because she was not close to me or anyone. She was missing emotions, and didn't talk to anyone about anything. It was humiliating. I was embarrassed that she would show up some place drunk. My father was enraged, he hit me, and that scared all of us."

Some families may not show these problems as openly. They may establish a facade of control and refinement in order to continue to deny problems with alcohol. This environment is also riddled with tension, strain, and trauma, but they are less visible because of the emphasis on control of thoughts, feelings, and behavior.

Some families recognize the chaos and trauma they have become accustomed to. Others only identify the chaos in retrospect. While they were in it, it seemed "just fine."

Tess Simpson, 15, whose mother has been abstinent for 28 months, says the drinking just seemed normal. She recalls that her mother carried a drink around with her, but Tess never thought about it. Then one day she noticed it, and saw it all the time from then on. Tess said her mother passed out on her birthday and Tess confronted her, told her she was drinking. After Tess named it, she knew she had been worried since she was 9.

Tess illustrates denial (Dorpat, 1985), an important defense mechanism in alcoholic families. Denial, which can operate at perceptual, cognitive, and affective levels, is a powerful refutation of reality. Denial says, "This does not exist; it's not true; it's not happening and it's not real."

Tess says that she never noticed that her mother always had a drink, partly because it was "normal." Either Tess got used to it or it had always been this way, so she did not consciously register her perception of the glass in her mother's hand. Yet she also "knew" it was there. She'd been thinking about it since she was 9. Until she became aware of the drink, she could not name it or give it meaning. You have to see it first to think about what it means. Or it can be the reverse: we know what something means, which is unbearable or unacceptable, so we block it out.

Until Tess could name what she knew was there, she could not connect her feelings to the glass in her mother's hand and to the chronic drinking the glass actually represented. Tess always believed that her stomachaches, fear, and deep disappointment were "in her head," made up because she was a "sensitive" child. Not until the family was in recovery and everyone was allowed and encouraged to talk about what happened during the drinking could Tess make the connection between her physical pains and the realities of drinking she was denying. In a drinking family, the therapist would be helping to make this link much earlier, challenging parental denial and distortion. Even without family recovery, Tess might have been able to speak about drinking if she had had access to therapy or supportive others who could tolerate hearing what Tess needed to say.

Tess tells us that one day she saw it and from then on she saw it all the time. She no longer denied her perception. She also put words and meaning to it, confronting her mother about her drinking. And then her feelings came: fear, disappointment, anger.

A therapist working with Tess makes a mental note that cognitive awareness came first. Tess could perceive the drinking and then name it. Her feelings came later. In some cases, affect comes first; individuals feel depressed or anxious, for example, and don't know why. The therapist helps the individual link the feeling to cognitive and perceptual awareness.

To outsiders, who often can see more clearly than family, denial can be utterly amazing because it is such a distortion of reality. But denial is also insidious. Family members, relatives, friends, coworkers . . . and therapists can all jump on the denial bandwagon agreeing not to see, not to name, and not to feel anything connected to the realities of drinking.

Why do people go along with this? Because the human need for attachment—a deep, emotional connection with others—is so fundamental it overrides everything else. People will readily sacrifice their wishes and views of reality in order to maintain a close relationship (Brown, 1988), or the illusion of closeness, or to ward off the threat of loss and abandonment.

That is also true of the family as a whole. People will go to great lengths to deny and distort whichever truths might threaten their security. Many people in alcoholic families believe that seeing and naming the reality will destroy the family, or at the least, they will feel disloyal and therefore guilty.

Ellie Barker, 7 years sober, her husband, Scott, and their grown son, Les, describe the chaos and thinking distortions, including denial, that were natural to all of them. It has taken them years in recovery to realize that such confusion, fragmentation, unpredictability, and inconsistency are not perfectly normal. Ellie says she never realized the impact her drinking had on everyone. She knew she was unhappy, she believed that was the problem, and she went on thinking that she had her drinking "under control."

Les Barker, age 25, had similar ideas:

"I didn't know I spent a lot of time alone. I just did it. And I never made any connection that anything in our lives had anything to do with alcohol. She wasn't staggering around or passed out, so I didn't realize there was anything wrong. We all thought it was her personality—to be changing so often, to have so many moods. I learned to be careful and work around her."

The therapist makes a mental note that Les's inability to register the reality of drinking probably had a significant impact on his development, certainly in shaping his explanations of reality and his view of people. The therapist knows that over time Les will likely be challenging and revising his perceptions and beliefs as his recovery and his relationships with his recovering parents provide a corrective experience.

Scott Barker recalls that the impact of his wife's drinking was mixed:

"It had no effect at all, and it was gruesome. I was naive. She said she was only having 'a drink,' and I didn't realize that she never ran out. 'A drink' was close to a fifth. I got irritated because her thinking would go loopy, round and round, so it was frustrating to communicate. I saw that nothing worked—there was constant arguing, yelling, shrieking, screaming. Nothing was certain; nothing was predictable. We did nothing together because nothing was planned. The only stabilizing thing in our lives was the TV. It was always on."

And finally, Len Irving describes a cooperative drinking lifestyle that he and his wife, Jane, enjoyed for years. It was all normal:

"We both come from alcoholic families where even the dog was given a beer. Early in our relationship, I would compete with Jane about who could drink more. She was clearly winning, and my ego was hurt. So I stopped noticing; I didn't see it anymore. She got irrational and exploded. This felt strangely familiar. It's what we'd grown up with! Jane became unavailable. I learned we had to communicate before 10 o'clock, then it was before 9 o'clock, and then by supper. The kids would scatter—everyone was unavailable and in their separate hiding places. The good times and the good hours were fewer and fewer. I had few feelings. Most of the time I was a plastic shell, and then I'd explode periodically."

This is trauma. The family context became more and more dominated by the emotions, thoughts, and behaviors of alcoholism. With the ease of flicking off the lights, Len was in denial: he stopped noticing, and he didn't "come to" till years later.

In our examples, we have clear descriptions of the alcoholic environment, remembered by people who created this context, lived in it, reacted to it, and kept it going. These families, with years of recovery, again illustrate the power of the narrative. What was real and traumatic can be remembered, known fully, and integrated into present reality.

The therapist helps the family use the narrative to acknowledge the trauma, to name it explicitly, and to understand its implications in the present. The therapist serves as a witness to and "holder" of the reality as denial lifts.

THE ALCOHOLIC FAMILY SYSTEM

As we have emphasized repeatedly, the alcoholic family system is unhealthy. It grows more rigid and narrow as alcoholism progresses and the need for defense increases. Normal growth is stalled or halted completely. As we have seen for some families, drinking is just the way it has always been: alcoholism is normal. Other families start out healthy but lose ground as they become confused, out of control, chaotic, and disorganized in direct response to developing alcoholism. This is like an undertow. The family members can't hold their solid (healthy) ground, which gets eaten away and pulled from under them by drinking. But it's not just the drinking or the drinker. It's also the "fitting in" and adjusting that everyone does in response. The Baxters—Deb, sober for 17 years, and her husband, Ron—describe the process of becoming an alcoholic family:

DEB: It was insidious. My drinking developed slowly, and I hid it almost from the start. We drank socially quite a bit, but it didn't stand out in our group. It did stand out at home when I began to drink for reasons other than social ones. We had four kids under 5 years old, so I used alcohol and drugs to keep going. I was sleep deprived, overworked, and couldn't ask for help. Also, I had a chronic nerve injury and began to drink to ease the pain. It's only now in retrospect that any of this looks abnormal to me—paying so much attention to drinking and trying to control it, even then. I remember my boys watching me take out the sherry and saying to myself, "How am I hiding this if they're watching?"

Deb illustrates a complicated defensive process: she combines denial, or the false illusion that she is hiding her drinking, with an awareness of what she is doing. Holding two separate, different realities in consciousness at the same time is called "doubling" (Lifton, 1986).

DEB: (continuing) But I did nothing. I lived in two worlds: I drank all the time, openly, and believed that no one knew anything. I acted like a spy, sneaking around, hiding it and fooling no one. My world narrowed, and alcohol became the most important thing to me. Ron had a flexible schedule, so he reorganized the family around himself as the primary parent. He believed it was his job to teach the kids to be independent and he set out to do so. Eventually I was ignored.

RON: I was a case of classic denial. I didn't want my wife to be an alcoholic, so she wasn't one as far as I was concerned. I'm a manager, so my whole professional life was based on taking over and solving problems. I jumped into this. We functioned like a family with a chronic nerve injury, even though it was difficult to recognize Deb after a day of drinking.

It was hard to separate our family's adjustment to the nerve disorder from our adjustment to alcoholism. They just got melded together. We explained everything on the basis of her nerve injury. Alcohol was dominating, but we didn't know it. I reorganized my work and taught the kids to take responsibility for everything at home—they basically lost their mother as a parent. We lived according to one basic belief: Deb is sick, so we don't disturb her and we don't expect anything from her. We 'take care of her' by organizing around her and becoming independent.

By operating on this belief, the family adapted itself to being organized by deception and thus became an "alcoholic family."

The alcoholic dynamics—denying the reality of the drinking while explaining it at the same time—often necessitate secrets and even outright lying. Denial means not seeing, not hearing, not explaining events accurately. Deception rules as the glue of relationship, and deception orders the system that structures family function.

System mechanisms, including structure (rules, roles, rituals, boundaries, hierarchies) and process (communication), establish constancy, define the structure of the family, and permit predictable, patterned, and adaptive behavior.

In the alcoholic family, these system mechanisms are geared toward maintaining the drinking. They are restrictive and defensive in the service of maintaining an unhealthy status quo. Family development, which should be flexible and expansive, instead becomes a constricting adaptation to pathology. Defensive patterns become entrenched, protecting active alcoholism. The alcoholic grows worse, the family grows worse, and all members try harder to keep from going under. Everyone's best efforts to control the damage keep the drinking system going and make it worse.

These defensive mechanisms of the system will weaken or collapse on the way to abstinence and in recovery. The therapist assesses these mechanisms during the drinking in order to challenge the family about its organizing procedures and thus further weaken the system, but also to anticipate difficulties that the family will have in recovery. Because of the immediate vacuum in structure, family members will be instinctively drawn back to old beliefs and behaviors that gave a false sense of security and family balance. What are these mechanisms?

Rules

Many rules, mostly unspoken, are required to maintain the double bind that enwraps the alcoholic family: there is no alcoholism here, so do not see it, name it, or talk about it (Black, 1981). What is real and what organizes family life cannot be acknowledged. The degree to which this distortion dominates varies between families and is an important determinant of alcoholic systems pathology. In general, the more alcoholism dominates the family system and the more it has to be denied, the greater the distortions required. Family members learn what is necessary to keep the drinking system intact, regardless of the cost. Though usually not discussed, they know, for example, not to challenge the status quo—Dad always gets drunk on holidays, though no one can acknowledge that this is true; yet the holiday is purposefully organized to permit and even facilitate Dad's drinking. Charlotte Evans remembered that the holiday dinner hour was always scheduled late, supposedly to give out-of-town guests plenty of time to arrive— yet guests always came in the early afternoon. The late dinner gave everyone extra hours to drink. These beliefs foster and maintain alcohol as the central organizing principle.

In our research families we observed a pattern of rules that structured their drinking systems and maintained attachments. Repressive, suppressive and constricting, these rules included the following: (1) don't perceive; (2) don't name; (3) don't challenge; (4) don't upset; (5) don't ask for change. In the "do" column, we heard the following underlying proscriptions: (1) do rationalize, justify, deny, and make excuses; (2) do maintain the status quo without question.

Family rules have an added impact on family interactions, often serving to define boundaries (Minuchin, 1974) as to who participates in the family, and how and when. For example, an alcoholic may have a drinking "buddy" who is granted open access to the home: he may come anytime, call anytime, and exert a dominant influence on family function. Very soon in recovery, the therapist may be called on to help the family change its rules or set new, temporary ones that will support abstinence. In the example above, the drinking buddy will lose his privileges. Sometimes families can readily understand this; in other instances the therapist, in monitoring recovery programs, should recognize the unchanged status of the drinking buddy, point it out, help the family members decide how to deal with the issue, or help them explore their resistance to taking any action.

Roles

Rules are expressed and solidified through roles, ways of seeing, feeling, thinking and behaving that hold the family system together. Roles can be thought of as "jobs" or "functions" that keep a family working, for better or worse. In healthy families, roles are clear and serve a positive, enhancing purpose. Things work well. In unhealthy families roles are often unclear and work in reverse: they keep the pathology going. Sober for 9 years, Joe O'Leary recalls the realities of family life:

JOE: Our days were normal and we drank at night. I thought we were close, but now I see that our children adapted themselves to my alcoholism. Becky was heroic, trying constantly to name the alcoholism and get us help. We called her our "pet daughter." She jumped in as a substitute parent for both of us and the other children.

BECKY: I was the one who saw it all. I remember trying to figure out how to tell them what was wrong. I composed letters and begged them to get help. It just seemed like it was my job.

JOE: Another child got into trouble all the time, shifting our attention onto him and off of our drunken fights. I always believed that I was a victim of my wife's bad moods, demands, and greed. I played the victim role to the hilt: feeling sorry for myself allowed me to drink because of all I had to put up with.

Much has been written about role in relation to children of alcoholics. Claudia Black (1981) and Sharon Wegsheider (1981) described several roles that kids assume as ways of coping with parental alcoholism. These roles are quite broad and fit for adults as well as children. They also fit practically any interpersonal situation. We all occupy a "place" and hold a "job" in relationships and much of role behavior is necessary and healthy. Black defined three roles that, in the context of adaptation to alcoholism, are not so healthy; although people may hold one particular role most strongly, they usually are familiar with them all:

1. *The responsible child, the one who takes charge, who cares for needy parents and siblings.* This is Becky O'Leary, above, and Cary Corwin. Adults taking charge may very well be doing what they're supposed to be doing, at least in caring for children. However, adults may take on way too much in other ways, protecting a drinker who has abdicated responsibilities, for example.

2. *The adjuster, the child (or adult) who is on guard to rapidly accommodate behavior and thinking to whatever is required by each*

situation. Len Irving told us how he stopped noticing and changed everything to adapt to Jane's drinking.

3. *The placater, the child who tries very hard to please or to focus off whatever is happening.* Remember Sonia Warner, who said all she ever wanted from her mother was a hug. Before she stopped drinking, she used to chauffeur her mother to bars. That was the best she could get in the way of hugs: to join her mother as a drinking companion.

Wegsheider (1981) added four similar, overlapping types: the hero, the mascot, the lost child, and the scapegoat.

Roles often substitute for a healthy self. Individuals become the role they are playing. They feel lost, disloyal, or confused when they cannot function in this part or it is no longer valued. Roles in an alcoholic family help sustain pathology. Individuals who attempt to challenge the role or the system are often pressured to get back into character. That is, they are urged to resume denial and whatever false beliefs and identities are necessary to maintain the drinking system.

The therapist should assess the various roles in a drinking family, point them out in challenging denial, and anticipate trouble ahead in recovery as family members flounder without the security of a familiar role. Entry into abstinence challenges their sense of themselves and their feeling of belonging in the family. The roles that guaranteed valued inclusion in the drinking system will be problematic and even unacceptable in recovery. But most people, and especially children, do not have viable alternatives. The systems vacuum of Transition and Early Recovery is in large part a reflection of obsolete roles and rules, with no replacements yet possible.

During drinking the therapist should point out the roles that sustain the drinking system. The therapist may also suggest that it would likely be hard for anyone in the family to imagine being in recovery because so much of their lives have been geared to drinking. The therapist begins to ask what it would be like, what roles can everyone imagine, if and when the family is abstinent.

Rituals

In alcoholic families important rituals such as birthdays and Christmas often become linked to drinking (Wolin et al., 1979; Wolin &

Bennett, 1984). Adult children of alcoholics remember holiday time with mixed emotions that typically include sadness and anger. Times for celebration and family closeness were marked by drunkenness and its predictable disappointment, chaos, and loneliness. Drinking and its devastation can get worse at special times. Becky O'Leary recalls:

> "I gave up being excited about anything after Dad got drunk and passed out at my 10th birthday party. I cried myself to sleep that night."

Others recall similar wrenching experiences. The linking of ritual family occasions to drinking heightens the anguish, because the holiday or special event was supposed to be anticipated with excitement. Many adults remember giving up hope and giving up the thrill of anticipation of such occasions, because they usually brought disappointment, at the least, and often devastation and calamity. Lou Klein recalls:

> "Every summer it was the same thing. We'd plan a family vacation, the day would roll round, we'd even pack up the car, but I knew it just wasn't going to happen. Dad would explode about something at the last minute and then punish us all by canceling the trip. Each year we used to guess which one of us would get the blame."

Parents who are not drinking often feel the pain too. So many told us that they wanted desperately to make it different, make it better, but parties and special occasions got ruined.

Rituals are often passed from one generation to the next, consciously and unconsciously. An individual who comes from a drinking family with drinking rituals will re-create, adapt, and even seek a similar family as an adult (Steinglass et al., 1987; Wolin & Bennett, 1984). The therapist should assess such rituals during drinking and recovery. How central was drinking to family ritual? Which rituals remain? What is the impact of the loss of ritual on family identity and loyalty? The therapist may work directly to help families construct new meaningful rituals in recovery. One of the most important is the celebration of sobriety birthdays. Some families will embrace this occasion, which now symbolizes unity and loyalty, as a whole. In other families, the sobriety birthday highlights ongoing problems and animosity. For example, some may wonder why the alcoholic got all the attention during drinking and continues to be the object of praise in recovery.

A mother told us she recorded the lives of each of her children in scrapbooks, which she presented to them on their 21st birthdays. She maintained this ritual through drinking, several treatments, and 8 years of recovery, a practice that provided a strong bond with her children separate from the alcoholism that dominated family life.

In assessing rituals and their role, the therapist helps the family strengthen those that have bypassed drinking.

Boundaries and Hierarchies

In drinking families, boundaries and hierarchies are likely to be blurred, particularly as parent–child roles are inverted. Sometimes the relationship between spouses is lopsided: the alcoholic, abdicating responsibility, becomes a child, leaving a hostile mate to take over parenting everyone. Family members experience both intrusion and abandonment by alcoholic and coalcoholic parents. Parental authority may be dictatorial or undermined completely by the chaos in the environment and the system (Schmid, 1995; Brown, 1988, 1991a, 1991b, 1991c).

The most functional boundaries are semipermeable. Family members have comfortable access to the external world. There is an ease in movement between the home and the larger environment. When boundaries are too open, the organizational patterns of the family are blurred. The family is chaotic, confusing, unprotected, and vulnerable to intrusion (Steinglass et al., 1987). For example, in-laws may dominate and threaten the integrity of the family. Fragmented and disorganized alcoholic families may typify this pattern.

The closed system is another family type. With rigid boundaries, the family is closed to interactions with the outside world. New information, new people, and new beliefs are rejected. This rigidity ultimately affects all aspects of the system: rules become stricter, with violations being punished more harshly; roles become rote, robotic reenactments. This creation of a brittle, "controlaholic" system is often a direct response to the increased uncontrollability of the alcoholism.

The term "hierarchies" refers to structured lines of organization, which in families are usually generational (Steinglass et al., 1987). In alcoholic families the hierarchy is often confused and inverted, as children typically assume a more parental role and position. The therapist ought to anticipate that this confused hierarchy and role inversion will be problematic for everyone in recovery. Children of alcoholics may feel unimportant and demoted when parents begin to assume their appropriate responsibilities. In such cases, the therapist might explain the vacuum in role and hierarchy and help the family make immediate adjustments so that basic needs of the children will be addressed.

Communication

Communication patterns reflect, reinforce, and define the structure of the family. If the structures are designed to support denial and the continuation of drinking, communication patterns will of necessity become maladaptive. You can't talk about a reality that is not supposed to exist.

In a drinking family, communication is defensive. It is designed to deny reality—the alcoholism—and to avoid dealing with it, so it is likely to be muddy, unclear, and obscuring. People in alcoholic families often speak in code. One family referred to Dad's drunken state as "the situation."

What could be more confusing? People learn to communicate about the drinking while still denying that it exists. Naming makes it real. If you call it "the situation," you can go on for years and nobody has to have a problem with alcohol.

Becky O'Leary recalls:

"I didn't know what was happening. As I got older I was noticing it more but still had no idea what was going on. I knew he [Joe, her father] was drinking, but I didn't know why it was getting worse. I had tried to get them to do something when I was younger. Now I didn't talk at all, not to anyone. I kept things inside and felt very discouraged. Later, I realized what it was, after the wrecked cars. In high school I could name it to myself, though I couldn't say it out loud. Eventually, as they fought more, we—the kids—would say little things to each other, kind of testing the water, like 'Can you believe he's drinking and it's Christmas?' Still, no one would say, 'Dad's alcoholic.' "

Communication maintains drinking and the drinking system. Truth telling, open, spontaneous self-expression, and problem solving are all sacrificed. Nor does communication have a forward, flowing movement. People recall that they felt swallowed up, chewed up, or simply more disconnected as a result of family communication.

The therapist here can point out communication patterns, including the following: indirect messages; passive use of language; codes and euphemisms; use of scapegoating to maintain distance; hesitant speech; paucity of needs or wants expressed; use of anger to avoid intimacy; use of a crisis, invoking guilt or panic, to bring the system back in line.

The Alcoholic Couple System

The dynamics of the alcoholic couple system operate just like the family system (Van Bree, 1995), but the focus of the members and the issues are often different. So we'll now highlight the two-person, adult relationship separately from the family with children.

As we know already, couples organize their relationship, consciously and/or unconsciously, to deny alcoholism and to explain why drinking is necessary at the same time. Before they had kids, Patti O'Leary believed that Joe needed to relax with drinks in the evening to unwind from the stress of his work and his unfair boss. She joined him each night for cocktails, which soon became an established ritual linking drinking and intimacy. In those days, Joe and Patti joked that it didn't matter where they were—if it was 5 o'clock, it was time for a drink. Later, when they had two small children, Patti replaced the unfair boss as the cause of Joe's troubles, becoming angry and demanding. According to both Joe and his wife, she was to blame for the radical rupture in their marriage. The trouble started when Patti wanted to shorten the cocktail hour in order to feed the children. He resisted, and she began to complain about his drinking.

Joe and Patti created a bond around shared drinking. Both "forgot" that Joe had trouble stopping each night, that he blacked out and couldn't remember their intimate conversations. It was Patti who suggested that Joe had a "sensitive" stomach in order to explain his morning hangovers. While still drinking cocktails herself, Patti began to feel isolated and lonely. Scared, she told herself not to feel this way, and then she didn't anymore. She replaced her dawning awareness of Joe's alcoholism with self-doubt and self-blame:

"I beat up on myself constantly. Why was I so intolerant and so angry all of a sudden? I tried not to be so demanding, sure that he would stop drinking if I shaped up."

Joe and Patti O'Leary believed their marriage was strong, close, and growing even though it was becoming increasingly organized around the need for alcohol and the distortions in belief, perception, and explanation required by both of them.

Many couples establish a social network of extended family and friends that drinks alcoholically and operates from the same distorted beliefs and perceptions. This wider group of shared denial and defense can sustain alcoholism for years or lifetimes. But if the social network does not drink alcoholically, couples will begin to have trouble relating to others outside their increasingly narrow and rigid system. With greater reliance on distortion, they have altered reality so much that they now live in a small, private world that others cannot share or challenge. The therapist points this out repeatedly.

The alcoholic couple's world grows narrower as both partners accommodate themselves to the distortions and demands of an alcoholic system. They may cease interactions with those outside, or they may live two lives, an inside world of alcoholism and an outside world of appearances, a different reality with different values and beliefs. The tension of maintaining the charade of two worlds and the fear of discovery prompt the couple toward greater isolation, which in turn makes it harder to reach for help later. Their connections are broken. Friends and relatives who do not support the drinking or the defenses of the drinking have been shut out or dropped. This pattern continues until one or the other partner steps out of the system. We saw that Patti O'Leary needed to leave the couple's drinking system when their children were born, a change that jarred the system and upset the balance of their relationship.

As we noted earlier, there is great variability in pattern, so that one family may appear quite different from another. That is why an individualized assessment is so important. What are the core elements that sustain denial in this family, at this time? Underneath these differences, the dominance and organizing influence of alcoholism are the same. For example, Fred Wiener realized that he and Callie were "an 'alcoholic couple' the day we met—I knew I was an alcoholic, but I didn't tell her and I pretended not to be for a long time." Fred had been in and out of treatment and recovery for many years. Drinking periodically when they met, Fred lived a double life for the next 7 years as Callie adjusted herself to the reality of his alcoholism, colluding with his denial, while neither one ever acknowledged that he drank.

Josie and Stan Moore established a different kind of couple system:

JOSIE: When I left college I replaced everything with alcohol. I was alcoholic when I met Stan. He drank very little with me so that drinking didn't bind us as a couple. But he liked me better when I drank, so alcohol brought us together. I got drunk constantly, and he didn't. We lived largely parallel lives without any real intimacy at all. We had the consequences of my alcoholism in our relationship, but neither one of us recognized the drinking.

STAN: My parents drank a lot, so this was nothing new. I lived in isolation, oblivious to Josie's drinking. I was in a lot of denial about everything in our relationship. The last few years I was sleepwalking, working more and more, and I wasn't in control of anything, though I thought I was. I was so dead, I liked her excitement and emotion when she drank.

INDIVIDUAL DEVELOPMENT

In the alcoholic system, individuals sacrifice their own emotional, physical, intellectual, or spiritual development to protect the drinking system (Brown, 1985, 1988, 1991c). Family members sacrifice their independent selves and the priority of their own well-being and development to preserve the couple or family system. To do this, such individuals must utilize psychological defenses that help them deny and rationalize reality, accept undeserved blame and responsibility, and project blame onto others. These defenses become so strong that they work like armor, a shield that some call a "false self" because people come to believe the distortions and to live them out. The real self, aware of reality, goes into hiding. Many people in recovery recall that "little voice" within that wouldn't quit, sounding the worry that drinking was the problem. Jane Irving (above) illustrates:

"I lived in a fantasy world which was completely real to me. I always believed my children and I had a very close relationship and we were a happy family. My daughter made a suicide attempt when she was 15. In her note she begged me to go to AA. I had no idea what she was talking about, and yet I knew exactly. The nagging voice in me had whispered AA quite a few times over the years. This was the beginning of a crack in my denial, but it took a lot longer."

As alcoholism progresses, others in the family must join this defensive system or live in constant tension because of the differences in belief and perceptions about reality. In the alcoholic family, individuals sacrifice their real selves and a realistic view of themselves and the world in order to maintain attachments and preserve the unhealthy drinking system. Let's now look at the individuals within the drinking family.

The Alcoholic in the Drinking Stage

As alcoholism develops, changes in drinking behavior and changes in thinking occur (Brown, 1985). The person experiences an increasing need for alcohol and a corresponding increase in the denial of that need. Two core beliefs organize the individual's view of self and the world:

"I am not an alcoholic."
"I can control my drinking."

In order to maintain these beliefs, the individual begins to exclude from awareness any information that might challenge them. This process of exclusion narrows the range of information the individual can acknowledge and builds the "defensive self." Eventually, the alcoholic is dominated by a web of distortion, deception and even lies. Harvey Thompson, sober for 6½ years, illustrates:

"I grew up drinking with my father and brothers. Drinking was what we did; everything evolved around it. There were times I overshot the mark, I'd feel guilty and have to apologize, but I had no idea drinking was the problem. Within a month of my marriage, Sue told me I was an alcoholic. I was furious. I became verbally abusive toward her, made jokes at her expense. My anger came out. She'd bring up my drinking, and I'd play it down and deny it. Sue tried to join in, but it nearly killed her and scared us both. I began to lie, to Sue and to my boss. Soon I couldn't tell the difference between the truth and the lies. It was important to me to buy the lies I told Sue. In order to make a lie work, I had to believe it."

The preoccupation with not being alcoholic and the focus on alcohol grow and eventually encompass the alcoholic's life. Relationships and activities not related to alcohol, such as church participation or association with nondrinking friends, are replaced by drinking activities and drinking friends.

The individual makes a "turn toward alcohol," the point at which the drinker ceases to choose alcohol freely and begins to need it. Harvey grew up in a family organized around his father's drinking. He and his brothers identified drinking with masculinity and with close male and family relationships. Harvey's "turn toward alcohol" was part of his early development. Others make that turn much later. Sue's challenge was the first time Harvey had ever paused to think about drinking, and at this point, 1 month into their marriage, he raged at her view of reality.

The need for alcohol is most often outside of awareness, which is why people have to create other reasons to drink. Members of AA recall with laughter that they drank to celebrate the sun coming up and they drank to celebrate its setting. There will always be a reason to drink, no matter what else may get in the way. Constructing the web of logic that makes drinking reasonable is the "alcoholic thinking disorder" that becomes the "defensive self" and the "defensive structure" of the family. The need to include more and more alcohol in one's daily life without disturbing the central belief in self-control becomes the organizing focus of the alcoholic.

Greg Hughes, sober for almost 3 years, gives us an example of a slower "turn toward alcohol":

"I drank in college, but I didn't really *begin* drinking till my 30s, when I began to depend on alcohol to relax. I'd been married for some time and, though we had always had problems, now they were related to drinking. We argued more, and I drank more to avoid the burden of everything. My drinking escalated as I felt deep shame and guilt. I couldn't fix my marriage, and I couldn't fix myself. This awful pattern slowly worsened over the years."

Rich Lawson, whom we met at the beginning of this chapter with his wife Molly, offers a final illustration:

"My drinking years started after my drug years. I had a minor scrape with the law and changed to alcohol. Initially I limited drinking to the weekends so I could pay attention to school. Then, when I graduated, my drinking escalated and I couldn't stop. I was barely 22 years old and I was there with addictive behavior.

"At first, drinking was OK and it was socially acceptable—more so than drugs. I liked the macho sense, the adventure. When I married we would 'go on adventures.' That was the code to go drinking.

"But then I began to have problems. I'd be brought home drunk, and my work production was down. I'd go to the office from 9:00 to 4:00 and get a bottle on the way home. I'd be asleep, or rather 'passed out' by 8:00, sleep till 3:00 A.M., and then prepare for work from 3:00 till morning. I organized my life to get in drinking. I went to different liquor stores because I didn't want people to know. I even bought chips and pretended I was giving a party. I threw them in the corner dumpster as I downed that first gulp.

"The home effect? I told my kids that drinking was a terrible vice, that I shouldn't do it, but I had to. I'd go to events but not participate. Our oldest child was the most shamed. I passed out in the car waiting to pick her up. Her soccer coach tried to wake me.

"Molly just cried a lot. Her father was an unhappy alcoholic who died shortly before we met. I was a partier, happy when I drank, which Molly loved. She joined me at first as we set out to 'have adventures' together."

The Coalcoholic in the Drinking Stage

In an alcoholic family system, the partner relinquishes initiative, accepts and contributes to the unrealistic view of reality and the turn toward alcohol, and organizes his or her life around drinking, just like the alcoholic (Jackson, 1954; Al-Anon, 1984; Brown, 1988, 1991c). The partner may join in the drinking or not. This reactive submission to the dominance of the drinker and the dominance of the alcoholic system is called "coalcoholism," or more commonly, "codependence." It ensures that one partner's developing alcoholism and the other's recognition of it will not disrupt their relationship or throw the marital system off balance as it did with Harvey and Sue Thompson, above.

The alcoholic partnership is like a dance: the alcoholic leads and the coalcoholic follows in a way that keeps them dancing. The leader may stumble, drift away, step all over the follower, or even break up the dance by changing partners. The coalcoholic's response is to try to keep the dance going.

Coalcoholics join the denial and distorted logic of the alcoholic in order to maintain an attachment and to gain an illusion of control and reassurance about the stability of the relationship. They become obsessed with the behavior of the alcoholic and preoccupied with the drinker's welfare. They may also feel ashamed and begin to close out the world, isolating the family further. The coalcoholic most likely feels fearful, insecure, powerless, and overwhelmed by low self-image and a sense of futility. The antidote to these bad feelings is to try harder to control the alcoholic, which only leads to failure. The coalcoholic sacrifices the priority of self-care, of being true to his or her "own self," attaching instead to the dominance of the alcoholic and the alcoholic system, which overwhelms the self.

While many partners join the defensive system with a hope of maintaining the marriage, Sue Thompson challenged the denial by naming Harvey's drinking a month after they were married:

"I thought I had married a stranger. Drinking became a means of separation between us. It didn't bring us closer the way it did with Harvey's friends. I didn't have the physical stamina to keep up once we were together all the time. I thought I had made a big mistake marrying and resigned myself to a distant marriage.

"But it was hard. His drinking escalated, and he became inconsistent. He denied and rationalized it all. I didn't want him to be an alcoholic, so I believed him.

"I still told him he was an alcoholic, but it was a long time before I really believed it. I took an evening shift at work so I wouldn't have to watch what he was doing. It was my way of shutting the blinds. I couldn't see so much of it and stay with him, but I needed to stay."

Here we see how Sue's need to maintain the bond required denial. She needed her husband and wanted to keep her family together, fundamental human needs and wishes. We also see her ability, in retrospect, to recognize her own needs and therefore her participation in the distorted relational pathology. Recognizing her own involvement has been essential to progressing in her own growth and to laying a foundation for an honest couple relationship:

> "I felt deeply disappointed when it finally hit me as true: Harvey was an alcoholic. His drinking was more important to him than I was. Everything evolved around it, and there was nothing I could do. It didn't change. I had a lot of fear. It was such a lonely feeling when I knew he was gone, that he wasn't part of a relationship with me. I didn't count, but it took me a long time to know it."

Recall that Molly Lawson, who chose Rich because he was a happy drinker, joined the denial and created an alcoholic system along with him:

> "I liked Rich because he was a go-getter—he had direction. He was controlling, but I liked that. I wanted to feel secure and taken care of. My father was a helpless alcoholic. We had a baby soon and were so busy I don't remember much about the drinking over the next 5 years. There was a bad undercurrent. I was upset a lot, but I always thought the next day would be better. We'd talk about it, but nothing changed and I'd blow it off. I kept control of myself by not drinking; he got worse.
>
> "Rich would go on binges, act bizarre, think bizarre. I got so confused. He told me I was mixed up, and I believed it. I felt like life had stopped. I felt out of control, and I defended him constantly.
>
> "We started in a big downward slide as he got into trouble. He had that awful motor accident—which gave me hope. We'd been through so much that I really believed he wouldn't drink anymore, but he did. I blew up. I got crazier and more out of control. I thought it had to be a nightmare, and I prayed no one would die."

Women coalcoholics tend to be more willing to accept responsibility and blame for problems in the marriage and for "causing" their husbands to drink. Coalcoholics confuse joining a drinking system or helping to create one, and thus contributing to pathology, with "causing" someone else to drink. They are not the same, though it takes a long time to understand this. Therapists know that the guilt this belief engenders is powerful and long lasting. Thus, they anticipate the reappearance of this view long into recovery and repeatedly challenge it.

The Children in the Drinking Stage

Children, like others in the family, adapt to their parents, their environment, and their particular family system. This process of adaptation is central to normal human development, in the context of a close relationship to parents or parental figures (Bowlby, 1980; Guidano & Liotti, 1983). Parents, along with the environment and family system they create, in turn shape the development of their children. Child development in an alcoholic family will be influenced and directly shaped by alcoholism—its environmental and systems aspects in concert with the parents' particular defenses and adaptations to the reality of alcoholism within the family (Brown, 1988, 1991a, 1991b, 1991c, 1995c). Much depends on the nature and degree of denial: what can be named and known about reality, and to what extent children can be protected or even diverted from the unhealthy developmental influence of parental drinking. Other people in the child's world are also important.

The therapist needs to know the answers to the following questions: Who was there? Who played an important direct, overt role in the child's life, and who served a more indirect, covert role that was nevertheless significant? Could any of these people acknowledge reality? Could they shield the child from the most negative influences of the drinking? Did they provide care, support, nurturance, and dialogue that bypassed drinking and was anchored in reality? In seeking this kind of information, we want to know how broad the child's world could be and how much of an alternative reality and life experience were available. For example, we know that many children of alcoholics view school as a refuge, a safe haven where (ideally, at least) there is structure, physical and emotional safety, and a focus on learning. This experience, so different from the unquestioned distortion and chaos at home, can provide reassurance and a sense of mastery that are essential for cognitive and emotional development to progress. Lyle Harding, told us he breathed a heavy sigh of relief as his father dropped him at school each day. He knew he'd be safe for the next 8 hours.

Some children tell us that they felt comfort and security with a sibling, a favorite neighbor, aunt, or camp counselor. Others recall sharing their sadness with the family dog, and one child, Tammy Curtiss, recalled the pleasure of her music lessons. She knew her piano teacher "knew," and so they "knew" together. Though they never talked about her mother's drinking, Tammy felt certain she was not alone.

In several of our research families, children were shielded by a nonalcoholic parent who actively protected them from being part of the drinking or experiencing its direct consequences. Betsy Jameson described two separate family scenarios depending on whether Roy, her husband, was drinking or abstinent. Home was alcohol free, so if Roy was on a binge, he left. Although their son, Tim, felt anxious as he sensed a binge coming, and abandoned when his father left to drink, his home environment and the family system did not change from not-drinking to drinking. When his dad was on a binge, his mom told him the truth and both talked about the reality of alcoholism. Betsy had been attending Al-Anon for several years, and urged Tim to attend Ala-Kid and Alateen, which he did. Betsy moved from coparent to single parent quickly, believing that it was important to hold herself and the family environment and system stable, with as little disruption as possible.

In the Harding family, initially Dad drank in the garage, believing that his children and wife knew nothing. Inside the home, he was a loving, involved father, so that much of the family's experience of him was positive. This double life worked until the effects of the drinking in the garage spilled over into the home. In the beginning, no one could explain Dad's sudden explosive anger at the dinner table or his need to go to bed at 7:00. Eventually, he spent more and more time in the garage and the other family members continued their lives without him. They all knew he drank: Mom couldn't talk about it; 14-year-old Sofie raged at her father, calling him a drunk; and 10-year-old Lyle increasingly stayed in his room, quiet and afraid. Eventually, the boundary between the garage drinking and the nondrinking home disappeared. With it went the sense of protection the children had felt inside the home.

In the interview we ask Lyle (now 15) what it is like to hear the family talk today. He says there is a lot of new stuff that he doesn't remember and there are things he recalls quite clearly: "I remember catching him drinking, and he yelled at me."

DAD: I drove Lyle to school every day, and a lot of the time I was wasted. I hit a bump, and Lyle hit his head and started crying. I shouted at the cat that had crossed in front of me, but there was no cat and we both knew it. I told Lyle not to tell his mother.

LYLE: It was tough because I had to cover it all up. I tried to forget a lot, and I tried not to believe what had happened, like getting yelled at. I locked myself in my room when my parents were fighting, and I tried to avoid Dad. I didn't want to believe that he drank.

Look how hard it is for a child to take in, to comprehend, to believe reality. Lyle wanted to trust and believe in his father. It is crushing to face the truth. A therapist working with Lyle or his family today could reflect back how hard it is to know the truth—then, and even now.

In other families, no one is protected and nothing is free of the influence of alcoholism. Sam Yarrow, whose mother has been sober for 12 years, recalls that his mother's drinking took up "all the space" when he was growing up. He continues:

"I think my first memory of her drinking was when we discovered her passed out in the yard. It was scary, but they [his parents] didn't say it was alcohol related. It was an isolated event. Then Mom started drinking late at night. I'd get up and discover her sitting alone with a bottle cradled in her arms. I didn't think much about it. I might have thought she didn't want me to see her. I didn't worry. It wasn't supposed to be an issue. I figured, 'It's not my business. I'm supposed to respect my parents, and I don't want to cause trouble.' I said to myself, 'Parents are good, parents will take care of me,' and I didn't see it anymore."

Here we see the turning point for Sam, the cementing of denial and the defensive "false" self (Winnicott, 1953). Since he had no alternatives to his parents' view and he needed his mom and dad (as all children need their parents), he stopped "seeing" what he was not supposed to see and he stopped "knowing" what shouldn't be known (Bowlby, 1985; Guidano & Liotti, 1983; Greenspan, 1979). It was too unsettling, even frightening, for him to continue to perceive what went on. And so he stopped registering the reality of his mother's drinking and increasingly strange and dangerous behavior. Sam continues:

> "Now I understand that Mom was drunk and she behaved strangely. I had a cough one time, and she gave me a cigarette to treat it. I thought that was weird. I did think, 'What's going on here?,' but I told myself that what happened wouldn't be important to the rest of my life. . . . I just told myself to be a part of this family and go with the flow."

Kids, just like everybody else, need to belong. They will sacrifice, just like everybody else, their view of reality, their feelings and perceptions, in order to feel "part of" their families. Most kids want their families to work, to be close, and to stay together. It is sometimes tragic what lengths we'll all go to to make this happen. Let's return to Sam:

> "You know, it wasn't until recovery that I realized how much was wrong. It's spooky finding out later on. When you're growing up with something, you consider it regular—this is the world I live in. It's scary to hear your parents wonder if they've raised you properly. You assume everything is fine when you're in it. Am I supposed to feel bad and worry now? I can't change the past. But I am beginning to wonder whether my tuned-out self was because of my environment. I always thought it was odd that I couldn't remember basic information about my family, like how old my sister was. I saw that my friends' families kept track of information."

We see that Sam couldn't remember basic facts because he was busy keeping his perceptions and feelings about unbearable truths outside of his awareness. Like Sam, many other kids living amid parental alcoholism often grow up feeling empty and even dead inside. So much has to be denied. In a way, denial is helpful too. It can be intolerable to really know the pain and hopelessness of reality if you can't do anything about it.

Although there are striking similarities in the experience of growing up with alcoholic parents, the particular pattern, the nature of attachments, the level of denial, and the degree of defensiveness and distortion required vary tremendously, as the above examples illustrate. It is thus important to look at both the similarities and the differences in understanding adaptation and development. It is also very important to determine the children's ages at the time the parent (or parents) became alcoholic, and whether both parents were alcoholic or, if not, which one was. Each child within a family will have his or her own "story" of "what it was like" growing up with parental alcoholism. Sometimes siblings will agree about the reality of alcoholism and family life, and sometimes they will wonder if they came from the same family.

In some of our research families, siblings were shocked to hear each other's memories and experiences. Some questioned their own recall immediately, believing that they must be wrong if someone else saw it differently. Others were more comfortable with differences in their perceptions and experiences, understanding that each person's reality was valid.

A child's view of reality is directly linked to the parents' view, especially if children are young. What a child can register as real and incorporate into his or her view of self and reality depends very much on the parents' view of reality and degree of defensiveness. Remember that children, in order to protect their attachment to their parents, will develop the same kind of "defensive" shell as their parents have. Sam Yarrow tells us that he stopped seeing his mother's drinking because he needed to trust her. And so he "tuned out" at a young age. In a family dominated by the environment and systems disturbances of alcoholism, "normal" development means an adaptation to pathology (Brown, 1988; van der Kolk et al., 1996; Krugman, 1987).

In an alcoholic family, the parent–child bond is usually structured to meet the needs and defenses of the parent(s) rather than the child. We saw Sam's efforts to reassure himself that his mother was OK, though his observations and feelings told him otherwise. The dominance of parental need leads to role reversal, rigidity, and confusion for children whose own development becomes skewed toward accommodation to others' wants. If family life and relationships are organized around denial and even outright lies, how is a child to go around this? It's only possible if there is someone willing to acknowledge a different reality.

As alcoholism grows more severe and more dominant in organizing the family, the child's development will be increasingly compromised. Sam shut down, repeatedly telling himself not to worry. In recovery, when the family began to discuss the realities of alcoholism, Sam felt scared. Hearing his mother describe how she drove drunk with several children in the car shocked him and challenged his denial.

Children develop defensively in alcoholic homes. They learn what to expect in the unpredictable environment. They learn to read the signals, whether these be physical or emotional, and they learn to react in predictable ways to keep the system in balance. They also acquire the roles and the view of themselves and reality that are necessary to maintain attachments to their increasingly distracted, distressed, and defensive parents.

The pervasive tension and chronic trauma of the alcoholic environment and system, as well as the traumatic, pathology-based attachment, cause all kinds of childhood problems such as anxiety, depression, and behavior disturbances. The children's world and the people in it are out of control, and the children can do nothing to change it. But they try.

Like their parents, children continue to adapt by doing more of the same—intensifying a particular role by becoming "more" perfect, "more" helpful, or even "more" disruptive in order to keep the system and their attachments stable. The children's feelings of anxiety, fear, and depression escalate, but they have no idea why. Eventually children internalize the chaos, confusion, inconsistency, and unpredictably that they have grown up with, developing deep problems with trust, the need for control, denial and distortion, concrete all-or-none thinking, and often a deep unyielding sense of responsibility for all that happened to them and to everybody else (Brown et al., 1989). Underneath their own defensive selves is an experience of profound helplessness.

Many adult children in our research reported the traumatic experience of mealtimes. Anxiety was pervasive, often the signal that fighting would soon break out. For many, mealtimes remain a trigger for anxiety to this day.

The greatest threat to family attachment and solidarity is the challenge of the family's denial about parental alcoholism. Children and adults will readily accept the secret keeping, joining the parents in the denial and distortion, in order to maintain family ties. Everyone in the family fears that telling the truth about drinking will result in loss of love, breakup of the family, and perhaps abandonment. The realities of the alcoholic environment and system take precedence over opportunities for healthy individual development. One of the most severe consequences of family alcoholism is the sacrifice of healthy development for both adults and children to the greater need of maintaining the drinking system.

CHALLENGES TO THE DRINKING SYSTEM

Movement toward recovery can begin when one partner "hits bottom," that is, when one partner can't sustain the denial and defenses any longer, or when something else gives way and someone in the family must reach outside for help. For example, the alcoholic or the partner may seek help for depression and begin to unravel the denial about the drinking, or a child may need outside help and drinking is recognized or even labeled. (But unfortunately, now and then, even though someone may seek outside help, the drinking is never mentioned or dealt with.)

When one partner seeks help outside the family, it changes the system, often for the worse in the beginning, because the status quo is disrupted with nothing to take its place. It also shifts the focus off of the system onto the individual who has sought assistance. Others in the family may feel so threatened by one person's seeking help that they pressure the "wayward" individual to rejoin the drinking system, literally giving up the "silly" idea that there is something wrong. Also implicit is the injunction to give up the focus on the self that is represented by this different view of reality. One of our research family members recalled being told she was "selfish" for seeking help.

Many families do not progress toward recovery even though someone has sought help, precisely because the threat is so great and things initially get worse, not better. Recall Sue and Harvey Thompson: She was shocked to see all the drinking she had managed not to see before their marriage. Only a month into being married, Sue reconciled herself to settling for a distant relationship and their couple system solidified including alcoholism. She could not join it, so she tried not to see it or to believe what she saw.

Sometimes a partner will attend Al-Anon or the alcoholic will try out AA, either of which will have a jarring effect on the system.

If the individual sustains the move outside and begins a recovery process, joining Al-Anon or AA, for example, or deepening a therapy process that identifies alcoholism, it will permanently alter the system. These families often experience tremendous discord, or certainly distance, as Sue illustrated. She became guarded as she actively identified her husband's drinking and attempted to disengage from a drinking couple system. Couples who stay together with such a split in their view of reality may end up living very separate lives. Or they may develop an angry, bitter, and accusing relationship—at war over what is real. Alternatively, the family may exist in peace and even satisfaction with two separate realities, as we saw with Betsy, Roy, and Tim Jameson, above. The drinking is acknowledged by one partner who practices a recovery program. Betsy altered family boundaries, requiring Roy to leave home to drink, which he did. Roy, by this time, responded well to Betsy's limits, as he had long been concerned about his drinking and wanted to preserve his marriage. He could respond to her increasing authority within the family, which she was learning in Al-Anon, before he could stop drinking. Betsy was in Al-Anon, living with an active alcoholic, for 4 years before Roy became abstinent and began AA.

The challenge to the system—someone seeks outside help—may settle into a new status quo, or it may move the family into the Transition stage, which we'll examine next.

CHAPTER NINE

Transition for
Couples and Families

Like a train barreling down the track, headed straight for impact with a mountainside, Transition involves the derailment, the crash, the convalescence for survivors, and the beginning of a new journey on another track.

Although it may not be quite as shattering as a train slamming into a mountainside, the move from drinking to abstinence will involve dramatic change. We often refer to this period as the beginning of the "trauma of recovery" because there is so much disruption and turmoil. Much of this process is painful and difficult, which makes it hard for anyone to trust that what is happening could be good for them or that it is a fundamental, necessary part of long-term health and recovery. As you read this chapter, reflect back to our introduction (Part I) when we said that "recovery is a good thing," that our families were unanimously grateful even though it had been an incredibly difficult and uncertain process leading to a kind and depth of change they could not have imagined. Most of this chapter focuses on how hard it is, on what it takes. As the researchers, we had the benefit and privilege of sharing with families as they looked back to remember "what happened" from the vantage point of their longer-term sobriety and family recovery. We could see Transition as part of a longer process. This gave us hope as we listened to their painful stories of the desperate, even cataclysmic, move toward the end of drinking and the unexpected shock of early abstinence. We had hope because we knew there was another side—the proverbial "light at the end of the tunnel," which they had come to tell us about. We urge you to keep that in mind now as you read. It's a very hard time, as the drinking family and the drinking world collapse and the foundation blocks for recovery are set in place.

It's a hard time for the therapist too. It is difficult to watch a family and/or the individuals in it experience such despair, which is necessary for "hitting bottom." The therapist may wisely seek support and consultation in working with families in Transition in order to maintain the longer perspective, to tolerate the distress, and to resist the impulse to reassure everyone that things will be OK. The therapist doesn't really know anymore than the family does that anything will ever be OK. The therapist does trust the process of recovery, however, if people can become engaged in it.

In terms of assessment, Transition is the period of the most radical change. As in critical periods in child development, in Transition certain tasks must occur for a healthy foundation to become secure. The therapist works toward understanding the components of denial— in essence, what core belief(s) must be protected—including factors in resistance and the meaning for the individuals and family of being alcoholic. The therapist listens for movement toward hitting bottom, and looks for vulnerabilities or openings in the environment, system, or within the individuals, where an interpretatation or challenge might be accepted.

For example, a patient has said she would know that she is an alcoholic if she disgraced and humiliated herself publicly. She has also told the therapist that she is not an alcoholic because she has never embarrassed herself this way. The therapist asks her what kinds of things she considers to be humiliating and points out how she has in fact done precisely what she fears. Moreover, the therapist notes that she has defined what an alcoholic is in a way that reassures her that she will not fit the criteria. In the process of wondering what it would take for her to consider herself an alcoholic, the therapist also wonders what would happen and what it would be like for her if she did.

In such a case the therapist must always be careful not to go so fast that the patient intensifies her defenses nor to go so slowly as to convey to the patient a lack of urgency in dealing with the seriousness and centrality of alcohol in her life. The therapist works on the premise (Weiss et al., 1986; Weiss, 1993) that the patient has an unconscious desire and plan to get well, which means facing the drinking eventually. Since the plan and the awareness of alcoholism are not yet conscious, the patient needs the therapist to recognize the realities of drinking and to "hold" this knowledge until the patient can literally catch up and accept it consciously. It does not help at all if the therapist colludes with the denial of the patient.

The therapist works to dismantle the defenses of the system, pointing out how rules, roles, rituals, boundaries, and hierarchies maintain drinking. The therapist can work with individuals, the couple, or the entire family to make repeated connections between the problems the family wants to solve and the drinking that maintains them. Like a broken record, the therapist plays it back: "The awful fights you have occur when you've both been drinking. You drink regularly, and you both think that drinking makes you closer. Yet you always end up arguing. What do you think this means? You tell yourselves and me that it has nothing to do with alcohol. I think it has everything to do with alcohol."

In the abstinent side of Transition, if all goes well the therapist shifts from challenge to direct support. The therapist helps build recovery structures, teaching about recovery and advising people to fill the vacuum of abstinence with external supports. The therapist recommends AA and Al-Anon directly if he or she hasn't done so already and explains why these programs are helpful. Having taken an AA and Al-Anon "history" earlier, the therapist now uses this information to anticipate and challenge continuing resistance to using these support networks. Or the therapist takes the history now: if people have been exposed to AA and Al-Anon, what was their experience, and if they have not yet been there, what do they think about going to these programs now?

The therapist continues to monitor recovery on all fronts, charting progress and watching for difficulties, including relapse signs, and any emotional or other problems that require attention. For example, one couple reports feeling depressed in the first 2 months of abstinence. The therapist helps them recognize that they both have felt a loss of alcohol and the loss of focus on their couple relationship. They then say that they have both reduced their support meetings to spend more time together. The therapist empathizes with their feelings of loss but quickly suggests that they return to their regular meeting schedule, reminding them of the tasks of Transition and reassuring them that they would have more time together up ahead. The therapist also asks if they feel comfortable sharing their recovery experiences with each other, noting that some couples find this very helpful and others do not.

In Transition, the therapist watches the developing process carefully and is quick to jump in, to explain what is happening and why, to anticipate derailments, and to help people get or stay on course.

OVERVIEW

In the drinking phase, cracks are beginning to form in the alcoholic system of rigid logic, rationalization, and behavior. The disadvantages and problems of drinking begin to outweigh the advantages. The individual suddenly begins to doubt the rationalizations or is presented with stark evidence of the centrality of alcohol that cannot be accommodated any longer. There is a tightening within the alcoholic family system. Everyone tries to keep the system from breaking down, which is paradoxical because everyone needs to give up, surrender to the reality of loss of control, and stop protecting the drinker. At the end of the drinking phase, the alcoholic hits bottom and decides to stop drinking, seeing no other alternative. Some family members may have arrived at this junction before the drinker, some may arrive at the same time, and some may lag behind. Ultimately, everyone needs to hit bottom, the "at-the-depths-of-the-soul" profound experience of helplessness and loss of control.

Following this surrender to reality, the alcoholic and his or her family can move into abstinence. Families often assume that once the alcoholic stops drinking there will be no more fighting, no more abuse, no more irresponsibility. They assume that abstinence will solve all the family's problems, since it was the drinking, in their view, that caused them. In fact, this newly abstinent phase is likely characterized by much of the same disordered behavior, illogic, confusion, and chaos. The only difference for most families is the absence of alcohol use. Paradoxically, the absence of alcohol uncovers tremendous problems that were hidden by the drinking; abstinence actually causes anxiety and stress, because no one yet knows how to behave or what to think in this new state. The unknown often feels frightening and much worse than the previous "knowns" of drinking or reacting to someone else's drinking. None of the old rules, roles, or responses fit anymore, but there are no automatic replacements. What feels automatic is a return to the familiar—the behaviors, thinking and relationship patterns that supported continued drinking. Instead of feeling confidence because of the "achievement" of abstinence, the alcoholic and his or her family feel powerless, confused, and ignorant about what in the world this all means and what in the world they are to do.

And this is what it's like when all goes *well*—because it is this experience of giving up, of helplessness, that forces people to reach outside the family and ask for help. If they are feeling confident about their "achievements," they likely will not reach out because they have not yet hit bottom—the acceptance of the inability to "have power over" oneself or anybody else. When family members discover that the problems continue or even worsen with abstinence, they may become angry, discouraged, and even despairing. They wanted to solve problems, not wallow in them or face new ones with no solution except "go to meetings, don't drink, and take 'one day at a time.' " The painful dilemma of Transition is how to accept the baffling and mysterious reality of "powerlessness" and build a new life around that acceptance.

The therapist here reassures the family members that this painful experience is normal, that they are not supposed to know what to do. The therapist supports the abstinent action steps they have taken and encourages them to listen in meetings and to attend a lot of them. If the family resists, the therapist might say, "It's hard to make sense of all this so soon, but it's not possible to go to too many meetings at this point. Let's look at the impact on the family and talk about what you can do to make this easier and support each other." Of course, the therapist is always making sure that children are protected and attended to.

At the core of AA and Al-Anon is an acceptance of loss of control. As individuals attach to 12-step programs and begin to reorganize their view of self and others around this philosophy, they are automatically guided to a focus on the self instead of on the partner or the couple and family. This is often frightening to all family members who believe that the help they need is to "put the family back together." Or they may expect help in learning "how to control" the drinking or the drinker. These individuals are still operating from active alcoholic thinking and an alcoholic family system that centers on trying to "get control" rather than accepting the loss of control. The therapist may directly explain this to the family.

In our view, the AA and Al-Anon programs are the optimal external sources of help, or "holding" environments, for the newly sober individual and family. These programs enable newly recovering people to refrain from acting out the old behaviors of drinking as they learn how to maintain abstinence and acquire the groundwork on which further change can build as recovery progresses. Before we move to the domains, let's look closely at Larry Macmillan, with 79 days of abstinence, and his wife, Corrine, who illustrate the turning points leading to abstinence and the baby steps of new recovery. Note how much detail of their history they both possess, even with less than 3 months abstinence. Often, the record of drinking, and even how people thought about it, falls into place once individuals accept the reality of alcoholism and its central organizing role. Larry and Corrine also illustrate how the recovery language and the framework of the narrative help contain impulse.

CORRINE: I think the first turning point came when we began drinking every night after work and we settled in to a regular routine of it. Neither one of us worried about this drinking until it got out of hand. We just kept doing it. Then Larry's father died and he started to drink alone.

LARRY: I was scared by her feelings about my dad's death, and I know I was scared about my own. I told her to snap out of it and she wouldn't, which scared me more. In my family you weren't supposed to cry; you hid your grief. I had to be on top of my feelings, and I did it by drinking. At least I had always done it before by drinking. But now I couldn't drink enough to maintain control of my feelings. I had to drink more and more, so I was constantly drunk.

The real turning point came when we went away for a weekend. I got drunk, and Corrine said, "How can you drink so much?" I said, "Because I'm an alcoholic."

CORRINE: I was scared and in denial. My parents were both alcoholics, so I couldn't take hearing this. I checked out and distanced myself from him. I never considered myself alcoholic, but now I'm thinking about it since Larry's been in treatment. The family meetings at the treatment center are very helpful to me.

We see Corrine taking in new information that will help loosen her denial about her own drinking. Larry illustrates the process of chipping away at denial as he let in information that would weaken his distorted beliefs and perceptions.

LARRY: The next turning point came for me when I let in the thought that something was wrong when I drank. I was drinking every day, and as soon as I got home I drank more. I got angry and enraged.

CORRINE: We had doozy fights. It was like putting gasoline on a fire.

LARRY: I thought I was drinking because we were fighting, but I had a secret fear that I was drinking like my father. He was an alcoholic, he drank every day and he was withdrawn. I always had a secret fear that I'd be like him.

I "hit bottom" on my last binge. I was gone for 3 days. I spent money, blacked out. I thought of myself as a better person than this, but I'm not. I lost control. I looked for more action, but I couldn't drink enough to quiet the pain.

I started going to AA meetings, but I hadn't really "hit bottom." I hadn't done any soul-searching, I'd had no treatment, and I had no "program." I didn't get immersed in any constant recovery. I thought, "I'll put my mind to it and just drop the drinking." It was not the case.

The therapist knows there is a difference between attending AA and participating in AA and hears that Larry was not invested in abstinence and recovery. Participating means becoming involved, getting a sponsor (for most people), and "working" a program. In charting attachment to recovery and the development of a "program," the therapist assesses engagement as distinct from attendance and points out the differences to the patient.

LARRY: A friend got killed in an accident, and I started drinking. Then I stopped and stayed dry for 6 months. I went to AA every now and then, checking it out. I thought, "I'm not that bad. I'll go back to being a social drinker."

Then I hit the end. I knew I was an alcoholic. I knew I couldn't control it. I was drinking constantly and couldn't still the pain inside. I just didn't have the power to control anything.

Now I'm a lot more vigilant. I watch out for triggers and am more honest with myself. If I think about having a drink, I have to do something immediately, like make a call or go to a meeting. I must not think I can "handle" this or get through it myself. And now I start talking too.

CORRINE: When he first started going to AA, we both had false expectations. We thought our marriage would be OK right then. We didn't know enough.

LARRY: (*wryly*) Yeah. No one told us about dry drunks.

The therapist chuckles with Larry. The "dry drunk" is the cognitive and affective state of drinking, now minus alcohol. Individuals may consciously crave a drink, or feel intensely dysphoric and begin to think about drinking. Now they act on these thoughts and feelings by calling a friend in AA and/or going to a meeting. They and the therapist know it is not time to sit with these feelings in an effort to understand them. This will come, even quickly, after recovery actions have been taken and abstinence is secure. In working with the Macmillans, the therapist might say, "Oh, tell me what's going on. What are you feeling and thinking? And is your program in place?"

CORRINE: We're very new, but we've been through enormous changes in almost 3 months. We have to learn to live without being enmeshed in the sickness, but we don't know what that's like. Now we just hear that it's possible.

Larry and Corrine continued talking about their adjustments over the 79 days of Larry's abstinence, illustrating the newly abstinent side of Transition. Both see the need to focus on themselves, pay attention to not drinking for Larry and to not trying to control Larry for Corrine. They illustrate the dawning awareness that they don't know much and what they thought they knew wasn't right and doesn't work.

The therapist hears this acknowledgment of "not knowing" as a positive sign and reinforces the AA guidelines of "one day at a time" and "first things first" by helping the couple to set priorities for maintaining abstinence.

This couple also illustrates that it is the behaviors of reaching out and taking new actions to substitute for the old ones that are primary. They have a beginning language of recovery from which to share their experience. The language also structures the uncovering process. Corrine says the idea of an "alcoholic family" is helpful to her because it explains a lot and helps her cope.

CORRINE: Yesterday I was talking with some confidence that wasn't cocky. But I really don't know what that looks like. I've still got a fear that something will happen, that something will screw it up. I'm doing things a day at a time.

LARRY: If I ask myself, "Will I ever drink again?" that's too big a question. I have to break it down and focus day to day. A few weeks ago we were struggling with our expectations of each other, thinking, "Now we can get our relationship back on track." Both of us can see it won't work that way. We don't know what will happen with us. The only thing I can say is "I won't drink today."

Larry and Corrine have an unusual level of acceptance and understanding of the process, particularly that they cannot seize control and manage it. The therapist knows that Transition is a time of intense assimilation and does not steer the couple toward problem solving unless something is in the way. This can be hard for therapists who do not feel they are doing their job if patients are not actively working on an "issue." In fact, the Macmillans are working to absorb new behaviors and thinking, radically altering old ways. If all goes well, the therapist simply coaches the couple to maintain their openness to being engaged in recovery and supports tabling what Corrine calls "triggers." In essence, the therapist says, "Don't work on the tough issues now if they're not interfering with recovery." (Many therapists might well scratch their heads at this "avoidance.")

CORRINE: The only thing I can say is "I won't leave today." I can't deal with issues of intimacy or communication, or make long-range plans.

LARRY: Talking about difficult things used to be a trigger to drink, so it's hard to do that now. We are accepting that it's OK to leave all the tough things alone for now.

CORRINE: There's a million little triggers out there, so we have to be careful. There's so much to learn without going into the triggers.

Larry and Corrine illustrate their intuitive awareness and anxiety about this new vulnerable state of abstinence. The therapist heeds their fear of taking in too much too soon, monitoring their behavioral and cognitive foundation building and supporting their caution about opening up difficult issues. The therapist knows that the focus now is primarily concrete.

THE ENVIRONMENT

Tension, despair, and hostility increase as the family members move toward a state of chronic inner and outer chaos. There may be more overt trauma, such as violent arguments. As the system is moving toward disruption and collapse, the environment may grow worse, with the atmosphere holding and expressing the fear and sense of impending doom that all are feeling and still trying to hide or stop. The environment is dominated by chaos, which may not be visible, and an absence of physical and emotional safety. Bad things happen, as Tanya and Steve Hoffman recall:

TANYA: I used marijuana, acid [LSD, lysergic acid diethylamide], mushrooms, cocaine—all in addition to my basic alcohol. I smoked marijuana around the clock from the time I was 16 till I stopped at 32. I smoked angel dust [phencyclidine] and sold it, but Quaaludes [methaqualone] were my favorite. I had a baby, and I would "come to" after functioning in a blackout. I had no idea I had a problem with anything.

STEVE: Our relationship was drugs and alcohol. Tanya wanted me to quit drinking or just drink beer, and I said, "Absolutely not."

TANYA: We got so we'd both swear off, but it wasn't for real with me. It was just something you said.

STEVE: I had a stopping point; I was a functional alcoholic. But I lost control of caring what I was doing. I got violent, picked fights verbally and physically. I would grab Tanya, be verbally abusive and threatening. Then I'd break things, slap her.

TANYA: Steve's version of violence was a fist in the face. My version was being grabbed till I bruised and choked. I provoked him. The bruises might be from me, throwing and breaking things.

Now mind you, we had children—the baby and kids from Steve's first marriage. They lived with all of this.

STEVE: My daughter died of an overdose, and I couldn't drink enough to blot out the pain. Alcohol and drugs stopped working. We weren't courageous. We didn't decide to quit. It all stopped working, and we came to a crashing halt.

The environment is chronic trauma. Each family member's life narrows to a predominant focus on alcohol, which organizes all of family life. Day-to-day living becomes less and less manageable and is marked by increasing failures and greater isolation. Children may be feeling more frightened as dangers increase.

Abstinence often comes after a calamity that traumatizes everyone, such as the death of Steve's daughter. Or it just comes, when the alcoholic hits bottom internally, or with pressure from the family's prior disengagement. Minus drinking, the environment remains apprehensive, dangerous, unpredictable, and inconsistent. The air literally hangs in a vacuum as people hold their breath waiting for something bad to end this state of dry alert. Some have described it as a war zone—after the last bombing—waiting for the next attack. No one knows anything about this new state, so family members stay vigilant and "walk on eggs," waiting for the alcoholic to drink while feeling certain that they will be the cause of it.

One of our families said that abstinence had produced an unexpected problem: the family had gotten so accustomed to living without Dad that it felt, quite simply, too crowded with him at home and involved.

If the family has reached outside for help, there may be some containment through advice from AA and Al-Anon members and/or treatment centers and therapists. Without external support and a framework to explain and reassure, the environment of Transition can be as frightening as the drinking. Pam Richardson describes the environment during the move from drinking to early abstinence:

"Matt always drank outside the home. That was normal life. But in the end, that boundary was broken. He drank at home and was drunk at home, which upset everything in our lives and scared us all to death. The kids were especially affected. They had so admired and loved their father. They had not seen or lived with him drunk until now. When their dad went to the hospital, the kids were angry and very resistant to the whole idea of 'alcoholism.' To them, it came from nowhere and suddenly the home was in complete chaos. Our youngest daughter kept saying everything would be OK if 'they' could just get me to stop crying. The kids blamed themselves. They've got worry in their blood. When we didn't know, when we denied Matt's alcoholism, we all believed we had a close, storybook family. The kids felt the truth destroyed their security and their positive view of their father. It was very, very difficult. They stayed furious with me for a long time. The oldest started using drugs right away. We got a lot of help in the first year, including family therapy and counseling for the kids. It took a long time for our family to come back to the closeness we had, or thought we had, when Matt was drinking."

Karen Graham remembers the environment with mixed feelings:

"There was a lot of fun and a lot of dark times. The atmosphere was dull; there's a cap on. We weren't real; we weren't as involved with the boys."

And finally, Jill Fitzgerald, describes her fears:

"I was so embarrassed and afraid my mom would show up drunk. She'd pick me up from the Scouts, and I'd just pray that Dad would be driving instead. Mom couldn't stay on the road. She'd drive up on the curb. She'd walk into the meeting and I'd turn pale—get out as fast as possible. It didn't change at all when she stopped drinking, except she wasn't drunk. I didn't see her because she was gone all the time. I remember feeling lonely for several years after recovery started."

All of these examples illustrate the dominance of chronic trauma in the context of family life in the move from drinking to abstinence. The disruption and uncertainty contribute to intense fear and an absence of safety. The therapist should assess the potential for physical danger and the need for active intervention to ensure safety. The therapist may also label this trauma for the family members and look for ways they can bypass the intensity of direct interaction. The therapist might explain that it is not necessary or helpful to try to deal with the couple's problems now unless physical safety is threatened. Children like Jill may need a lot of support, education, and substitute parents through this painful time.

THE SYSTEM

During the drinking phase of Transition, the tension is steadily building until one person "hits bottom." At that turning point, the individual chooses recovery and takes steps outside of the alcoholic family system. Whenever one person moves outside of the system, the entire system is altered. The Parkers illustrate a 10-year period of Transition, as one person after another left the alcoholic system and began a separate individual program of recovery. Peggy reports:

> "Our son Jeff was first. He was picked up by the police as a suspect in a gang attack. We readily accepted the label 'alcoholic' because it was better than 'criminal.' He went to treatment and began recovery. Everyone in the family reacted like someone had died."

The therapist takes note of the loss everyone experienced as one member stepped out of the system. Peggy continues:

> "Two years later, I reached my bottom. I had watched Jeff change, and my own denial began to erode. I got to the point I knew I was alcoholic and it was now OK to be one. Over the next 7 years we lived with two recovering alcoholics and two active alcoholics left."

During this evolutionary process of systems change, the family members lived with two versions of reality. Each person who entered recovery shifted priority from the family to themselves as individuals. Peggy says:

> "As my denial slowly lifted in recovery, I focused more and more on myself. This was good or I probably wouldn't have been able to leave my husband alone about his drinking. I could see the reality of alcoholism in my family. I knew it was hereditary. I knew I had been abused. I was letting all this in. I knew I was really in recovery when I told my husband he was no longer my first priority."

In the interview, we saw evidence of separation between the family members when Peggy's husband, Jared, disagreed with her recounting of events and she told him, "This is my story."

Nine months abstinent at the time of the interview, Jared had "joined" a family in which his wife and son were in Ongoing Recovery as individuals while the family had remained arrested in development. The family lived in the unchanging status quo of two different realities—a drinking scenario and system and a recovering story and system—over the same time period. In the last 9 months, the family system moved from two different versions of reality to one, as both parents were now identified in recovery and the family began a process of unified systems growth. Only one drinker remained outside this new system.

At the end of drinking, we emphasize again, the system is in a state of chaos and collapse that is uncomfortable, confusing, and frightening for everyone. But it is necessary and normal. Still, if family members have not hit bottom themselves, they are likely to try to hold the family together, resorting to the very patterns of behavior and beliefs that kept the drinking system going. It is indeed that intensification of efforts to control the system that ultimately leads it to collapse.

Most families remember significant "turning points," events or changes that shifted the system, facilitating the move toward abstinence, when no one was yet identifying alcoholism. These turning points become part of the narrative that people use in recovery to alert them to danger, such as the reemergence of old thinking or behaviors. Karen Graham illustrates:

"We drank wine together in the evenings for many years, and I couldn't see any problem. Then I went back to school for management training and I couldn't drink at night. Pretty soon, I was much more aware of Bill's drinking. We began to have problems, and he blamed my going back to work as the cause. I thought so too. It *was* the cause in a way because it opened the space for me to see Bill separately from me or from us as a couple enjoying each other's company in the evening."

Sheila Bryce recalls the major event that jet-propelled the engines of change for her mother and father:

"Our family always drank, and none of us ever saw it as a problem. Our friends' parents drank, so we grew up with alcohol as a normal part of daily life. In the summers, our home was a gathering spot for neighborhood social life and drinking just flowed. Then my mom got cancer. That was like a bomb. Her doctor told her she needed to reduce the stress in her life if she wanted to survive, and she came home and told my dad he had to quit drinking or she'd leave him. They'd been married over 30 years! And nobody had ever mentioned drinking as a problem!"

This family, the Bryces, catapulted into abstinence. Dad entered a treatment program immediately and remained abstinent. Mom and Dad went to AA and Al-Anon for a brief time and then decided to be in recovery "as a couple," supporting each other, which we think, lowered their opportunity to focus on individual growth. They stabilized as a "dry" system, but not one that could easily change.

A therapist following them in recovery would actively challenge their decision to stop attending meetings and ask them why they needed to do this now. Frequently, one or both partners feels threatened by the loss of a drinking symbiosis, which can be reinstated if both partners stop their outside help. The therapist would need to offer additional support for the separation, reassuring them that they can be a "recovering couple" by supporting each other in their separate programs. If they continued to resist, the therapist would question what was standing in the way. One partner might be drinking and want the other one to start again, or one partner might not feel able to establish a recovery focus on the self and so would need the partner to give up the individuation of recovery by refocusing attention on the dyad.

Another couple illustrates the absence of systems change early on. With 5 months of abstinence, Marissa Morgan felt excited about being in recovery and very anxious at the same time. When she talked about herself as an individual in recovery, she was clear in her language and calm emotionally. When she talked about herself within the marital relationship, she became so confused and agitated that she could not follow a logical progression. It was clear that her alcoholism had been an important part of the couple bond, a partnership that her recovery had threatened severely. Mort, her husband, had sought no help and had no program of recovery. While he supported her abstinence verbally, in the interview he "dropped out" emotionally when she talked about it, fidgeting and looking away till she returned to talk about him and their marriage. Like many similar couples, Marissa wanted Mort to find a program for himself, in part so she could feel less guilty about focusing her attention on herself instead of him.

Marissa illustrates the difficulties for partners when only one is in a 12-step or other kind of recovery program, our Type II couple. AA or Al-Anon may be viewed as an intruder, the third point of what is now a triangle. Many non-12-step individuals say they felt as if the partner was having an affair—going to meetings and out for coffee, talking on the phone. What about the couple? It's terribly hard to understand that the newly recovering person has lots of time for 12-step friends but no time for the couple.

The therapist empathizes with both partners about how hard this is and also explains that it is normal. The therapist wonders (again) if the partner has been to AA or Al-Anon and explains why it is important to go. The therapist does not help the couple solve the disruption to their bond by facilitating work on "the relationship." The therapist does help them make adjustments so they can better tolerate the turmoil. Beyond explaining what is normal, the therapist helps the couple tolerate the vacuum so they do not need to impulsively restore the old system.

In the abstinent phase of Transition, the newly dry family is in a state of crisis. Even though the Drinking stage had a lot of problems, it also had its own equilibrium, which has now been thrown into pandemonium. There are many possible scenarios for new abstinence. The alcoholic may be viewed as "good" for facing the drinking and stopping. Yet family members may also experience a barrage of feelings of bitterness, resentment, and anger toward the alcoholic for all the negative behavior they have tolerated and adapted themselves to in the past.

Alternatively, family members may feel relief that the drinking has ended and fear about facing interpersonal problems. They believe that addressing these issues might cause the alcoholic to drink or might force other family members to face themselves more quickly than they are able to. It is common for the family to feel anxiety and confusion about how to communicate and problem solve regarding everyday business and deeper emotional difficulties. One man said he and his wife agreed not to talk with each other about anything in the first year without first checking with their sponsors. While this sounds extreme to many who value a return to the couple focus as soon as possible, this couple found it a very helpful protection. They weren't ready to communicate without help. Inserting the buffer of sponsors between them also kept their couple focus to a minimum as they both invested all their time and energy in their individual recoveries. They told us it was a 10-year process of becoming completely open in communicating with each other. By that time, they had a different couple system in place, one which gave them a foundation of new rules, roles, and boundaries that enabled them to communicate effectively as equal partners. Couples cannot decide to "be equal." They grow into it as they and their marital system increasingly tolerate individual autonomy and development. This tolerance for separation is the foundation for a new couple system. Unfortunately, many couples end their relationship before reaching this point of new possibility.

Couples may end their relationship for several reasons. Some couples believe that any good will and love was eroded away by the drinking. They see no purpose to keeping the relationship going in this difficult time of Transition. One spouse may be in recovery and the other is not. Frequently, women entering recovery are left by their husbands. Or too much emphasis and stress is placed on the couple system at this stage. Partners simply aren't capable of improving their relationship at this point.

As we've already stated, when both parents organize themselves around AA and Al-Anon, the family benefits from the external support of shared new beliefs, values, and attitudes about alcoholism. They will establish a common bond, and share new behaviors and a new language that can hold them on similar, parallel recovery paths.

As a result of the chaos and increased anxiety, everyone in the family is vulnerable to developing a range of symptoms and problems during this stage. Addictive disorders such as overeating, smoking, or alcohol and drug use may emerge or intensify. Spouses may abuse prescription pills. Children may act out their feelings of fear and confusion as a way of taking the focus off the alcoholic. Anyone may develop acute depression or anxiety. One of the spouses may decide to end the marriage or have an affair. All of these reactions to the radical change of abstinence are common. It is hard to sit still and watch the system collapse. It is also hard to ask for help. With the drinking system's collapse, the family faces a void. Abstinence was supposed to solve the family's problems, but instead it ushers in a frightening vacuum. Systems growth is still down the road. Pam Richardson recalls:

"In the early years, Matt's alcoholism was outside of the family. He lived two lives, a drinker in the world and a family man and good husband and father at home. We were not an alcoholic family, except in the way we accommodated to his time away. But it wasn't a lot different from other families where the dad was gone a lot at work or traveling and the mom raised the kids. When our world collapsed and he went into treatment, we became an 'alcoholic family' immediately and it was very hard. We had to challenge our view of everything. We didn't come into recovery with a painful history of alcoholism, yet this is what we were and what we had to face."

Pam told us she did not hit bottom herself because of Matt's drinking: she discovered that he had been having an affair, and it was that severe shock that pushed her into seeking help.

With the collapse of the unhealthy drinking system, the family's rules, roles, regulatory processes, and rituals do not work. For example, during the drinking, the coalcoholic may have covered for the alcoholic at work, a behavior that becomes unacceptable in recovery. The coalcoholic's new behavior—refusing to protect the alcoholic—alters the family system, an adjustment that everyone may find painful in the beginning. In addition, a family's rules such as "don't trust" will be challenged as family members slowly grow to trust the recovering alcoholic or coalcoholic and as they learn to focus on and trust themselves. However, the beginning process of developing trust is uncomfortable and scary for all.

Family rituals that used to revolve around drinking, such as a parent predictably drinking heavily on the weekend and therefore not keeping any promises regarding activities with the children, will be replaced by unstructured time, which will be filled by attendance at meetings. Roles are now, or eventually, shifted, with parents functioning as parents. This adjustment relieves children of the inappropriate parenting responsibilities they carried. While this rearranging and restructuring of roles is very positive in the long run, it may be awkward and uncomfortable early on. Ironically, children may feel more frightened letting go of the parental role when they don't trust their parents to be competent to take over.

Each person in the family needs support while the family is so unstable. Parents need to focus on themselves, which they accomplish by reaching outside the family. But they also must pay attention to their children, which is very difficult to do. Many parents sacrificed parenting responsibilities during the drinking, so they do not have parenting skills to draw upon. Ironically, and unfortunately, they also may now become *less* available to their children because of the need to put the attention on themselves. Many family members comment sadly that recovery meant more loss and abandonment during Transition than during the Drinking stage. Tanya Hoffman explains:

> "This was really hard for me. My son had been devastated by my alcoholism, and I'd been at home. Now I was told to 'do 90 in 90' [the recommendation that newcomers go to an AA or Al-Anon meeting every day for 3 months], and I felt like I was using my son as an excuse not to go so often. I have a problem with anyone telling a mother to abandon her children twice—once to alcohol and again to AA. I completely abandoned my child to my own need to be in AA and to be so self-absorbed. My big regret now is that I owe my son for recovery as much as I do for drinking."

Children *always* need parental attention and support. When they cannot have it, as sometimes happens during the trauma of Transition, it is absolutely necessary to provide substitute caretakers and outside support. Children's programs that are affiliated with addiction treatment centers can be very helpful, as well as counseling and therapy. It is our hope that childcare will become intrinsic to treatment and readily available in all communities. Families should not be faced with a choice of being in recovery *or* parenting their children, which is how Tanya felt.

THE COUPLE IN THE TRANSITION STAGE

The collapse of the alcoholic couple system provides an opening for help from outsiders in rebuilding the faulty structure. The crisis of the end of drinking and the exposed vulnerability and intense need for help that surface in the wake of abstinence permit both partners to avail themselves of the protection and guidance of outside supports.

As the couple enters recovery via a treatment program, therapist, and/or AA and Al-Anon, they both suspend their focus on the relationship and move away from each other and the bond they shared based on the denial of alcoholism. The "holding" environment of the 12-step programs functions like a substitute family. In treatment, they are coached to take the focus off their mate and off the problematic ways of relating within the relationship and to focus on the self instead. Ron Baxter, whom we met in Chapter 8, illustrates:

"I felt shocked and abandoned when my wife went into recovery. I wanted to be supportive, but I had no idea how or what that would be. I felt afraid and sensed a huge split between us. I had one appointment with my wife's therapist, who told me bluntly to find a program of recovery for myself. The therapist said, 'Go to Al-Anon.' I did. We began a process of putting our lives back together around common values. We both committed ourselves to recovery, which is not the same as committing to each other. That couldn't come till later."

Deb Baxter was philosophical as she recalled that the first few months were a "time-out" for the couple:

"There was an absence of communication, not a breakdown. I realized it just wasn't there. I had trust that our adjustment together would come down the line. He had to focus on his recovery. I didn't delude myself that everything was worked out. We'd get to the other stuff if it was worth getting to. But I wasn't in a hurry. Things were working at the moment."

Deb actually welcomed the "pause" in couple focus once she felt reassured by her therapist and recovery friends that it was normal.

The 12-step program offers couples a structure they desperately need. In the beginning, the alcoholic and coalcoholic may totally immerse themselves in the recovery world. The language, literature, and socializing may constitute the whole of a couple's life, and most of this will be as separate individuals. They may feel as much or more emotional distance between them as they experienced during the drinking. This time, however, the work they are doing individually will allow them to work toward a more satisfying couple relationship in the long run.

Let's clarify something about the element of time at this juncture: "short-term" recovery is not "full-term" recovery, and "short-term" sobriety is not the end; "short-term" (Transition) is a window, a piece of the whole. When couples are encouraged to put the focus on themselves as individuals and *not* to try to "fix" their damaged rela-tionship during Transition, this is not forever. Yet, because people cannot see ahead, or even imagine what a healthy couple relationship might be like, they are afraid that this shift in focus will lead to the end of their bond. That sometimes happens. But just as often the failure to let the couple system rest, to let it wait in collapse, leads to the end of relationships as individuals feel cornered and forced to choose between their recovery *or* their marriage. Marissa Morgan, above, demonstrated this dilemma. She could not talk about her marriage without becoming confused. Her vocabulary became murky and vague, as she obscured reality for herself and her husband. Both Marissa and Mort were terrified that her recovery and the absence of his would draw them apart.

Another couple, Denise and Tony Castle, decided to "separate" on the advice of counselors in the treatment center. They both understood that this meant "emotional" separation. They needed distance without cutting ties. Denise laughingly tells us what they did:

"We needed to separate physically, and we would have if we could have afforded it. We just needed space. I was so angry and not at all ready to forgive and continue living together as if nothing had happened. And I didn't want to be nice and understanding. We made a 'separation contract'—we would live for the next 6 months 'as if' we were not a couple, though we'd continue in the same house. It would be like roommates. This gave us freedom to go our separate ways and attend to our separate needs in our programs without worrying about the other."

The interviewer asks for more details about the living arrangements. How did they actually stay separate? Was the interviewer correct in assuming they had separate bedrooms?

Both Tony and Denise chuckled warmly as they looked back from 9 years of recovery—they changed nothing. Tony said they continued sleeping in the same bed, but they faced opposite directions. Everyone laughed.

Karen and Bill Graham (above) provide another example of "turning over" to an external authority: "We made an agreement to do everything the treatment center recommended. It helped us immensely because we stopped fighting."

Several of our research couples could not make the move to an external authority. They continued to rely on each other, or one relied on the other, in a parent–child way instead of reaching out. In all cases, depending on each other for recovery stalled individual development as the couple relationship and system continued to take priority over individual development. The couples remained enmeshed around abstinence in the same way they had been enmeshed around drinking.

Tina and Danny Zlotnik both saw that he was the one who had power and self-control. He was the strong one, the protector. He would keep her sober. Both accepted Danny as Tina's "external authority" or "higher power." The therapist wonders how they arrived at this agreement and how it serves them. Then the therapist asks how it doesn't work.

At an unconscious level, Tina and Danny know that no one, including him, AA friends, or sponsors can do it for her. But according to Danny: "Tina will never have to drink again as long as I support her and I am in control." Danny was upset, however, when Tina became depressed and he realized he did not have the power to make her feel better.

The therapist hears that Danny has not faced his own powerlessness. Until he accepts that he cannot save Tina, the couple system cannot change from its current parent–child structure to a more equal system based on individual autonomy. A therapist would continue to investigate how this system serves Tina and Danny so that they cannot give it up.

Another couple illustrates a similar dilemma. Toby Grant stopped drinking and that was the end of it. He utilized no outside supports of any kind. He wanted his alcoholism to be in the past, over and done with. He did not want to have a "story" of himself as an alcoholic, and he didn't want to talk about it. He wanted to get on with his life and focus on building a closer relationship with his wife, Janet.

In essence, Toby wanted to split off the out-of-control part of himself, a psychological defensive process that will create new problems for him and the couple. We can expect Toby to experience dissociative symptoms and to feel empty in abstinence as a result of shutting out the past. If Toby could focus on himself and construct a narrative, he would likely experience tremendous pain as he integrated the realities of the past into his growing sense of himself in recovery. We know that his childhood with alcoholic parents was one source of his wish to deny the reality of his own drinking.

Janet has had trouble with his wish to shut the door. She tells us she was left hanging by Toby's erasure of his past because it wasn't just "his past" but her past, too. She needed to be able to talk about what had happened between them with his drinking and his being an alcoholic.

She recognizes that his reluctance to acknowledge the past pushed her into denying it too, which paradoxically kept them both locked in the past.

TOBY: I don't think about it, although sometimes I wonder if I might be preserving the old system. But there's nothing to talk about on the surface. I am puzzled when Janet thanks me for not drinking.

JANET: (*responding*) I'm bottled up because you don't think about it.

She knows unconsciously that she is carrying knowledge and feelings for both of them, a container function she doesn't want. Janet knows she needs to talk, but she thinks it has to be with Toby. She has no idea why she has never been to Al-Anon, and she is surprised to learn she can go there even if Toby doesn't go to AA. If Janet goes to Al-Anon, which we have recommended, it will automatically alter the system.

A final example offers another illustration of a partner's continued distorted thinking: "If I focus on myself, it will undermine the couple relationship. All the focus will be on 'me' instead of 'we.' " Exactly right. For the short term, this is very helpful. When the separation has been accomplished and both partners are focusing on themselves, they can often come together sooner rather than later. The therapist can say this directly to the couple.

Hillary Raeburn describes it:

"I was upset. My husband's sobriety was first, and all he did was go to meetings. He had serenity, and I needed some. I went to a 1-week family program, and I learned about alcoholism in our family and in my own first family. From then on, we drove to aftercare together every week. I went to my meeting and focused on myself. He went to his and did the same. That time was a bridge back to our couple relationship because we started communicating. Since we were driving to and from recovery meetings, that's what we talked about. It was a good foundation."

INDIVIDUAL DEVELOPMENT

The Alcoholic in the Transition Stage

The Transition phase is characterized behaviorally by the shift from drinking to abstinence. The disadvantages and problems of drinking begin to outweigh the advantages. The defensive thinking that kept it all in place begins to crack. As denial erodes, the alcoholic begins to experience despair, loss, failure, and an increasing isolation. Irene Cooper recalls:

> "I went to AA meetings for 4 years before I stopped. I had started to worry about my drinking, and I was afraid of all the 'yets' I heard in meetings. It was hard. I wasn't ready to stop drinking, but I hoped to avoid all the awful things I knew were ahead of me. Being in meetings made me scared and I hated it, but it was the only place I heard reality. My world wasn't collapsing and people weren't challenging me about anything."

The feelings of despair and defeat are essential to the recovery process as they keep the alcoholic moving toward the point of hitting bottom. Many individuals describe a process of "fits and starts" (Bean, 1975a, 1975b) during Transition as they oscillate between degradation and despair, on the one hand, and a resurgence of hope, even inflated grandiosity that "I can control this thing," on the other. Many go back and forth between drinking and abstinence as they struggle to hold onto the belief in loss of control, reach outside themselves for help, and embrace abstinence. Again, our research families told us how very difficult it was to maintain these deep internal changes without support. Many note that their early rejection of AA stemmed from the horror of accepting loss of control and their willful, determined stance to do it on their own. Harry Quinlan remembers:

> "It's ironic; I hated dependency and dependent people. I believed in self-sufficiency and the old 'bootstraps' philosophy—you pick yourself up and get control. All the while, I was completely dependent on alcohol and believed I needed no one."

When the alcoholic hits bottom, the next step is surrender, the acceptance of loss of control of drinking. The individual moves from the beliefs "I am not an alcoholic; I can control my drinking" to "I am an alcoholic; I cannot control my drinking."

Harvey Thompson (from Chapter 8) remembers the awful downward fall:

"I was desperate with the baby coming. I told myself repeatedly it was time to stop drinking and using drugs; that I couldn't be a father and keep doing what I was doing. I was filled with terror. I lived in a fantasy world, telling myself and Sue that I was going to quit, but I never made it. Each time I'd make the promise, it was more of a disappointment. I was a guy who'd had self-confidence, and I was losing it.

"I stopped promising for a while. Then I set up challenges: If I ever drink and use dope at work, then I'll know I have a problem. I did. If I ever drink and use dope when I have a business meeting, then I'll know I have a problem. I did. If I ever drink and use dope when I have to drive, then I'll know I have a problem. I did. I couldn't make any of my goals, and I just kept stuffing the painful awareness of my total loss of control."

As long as the risk of taking a drink is present, which is primary during Transition, the alcoholic needs to substitute other actions in its place. For instance, individuals substitute a walk or an AA meeting for the cocktail hour. When they feel a craving to drink, they act on it with a phone call to an AA friend or sponsor. It is necessary to maintain a sharp, vigilant focus on alcohol during this time. The therapist can help by keeping this focus in place or wondering why it's not.

New abstinence in Transition is an acute, crisis period. It is all about action—acting on new abstinent behaviors—and new thinking, especially the constant reminder, "I am an alcoholic." Individuals need to maintain abstinence, which they do not know how to do. The act of taking a drink has been automatic.

In addition to new abstinent actions, which is "staying dry," much of the focus in Transition is on adjustments to "being dry." Some people say that new abstinence feels like a foreign land or a strange new coat that doesn't fit. Irene Cooper (above) describes it:

"Alcohol is as much a part of my life now as it was during drinking, except in reverse: I'm not using it. What I mean is how much I have to think about it. I think about it *all* the time. I'm scared not to think about it. I have to think about simple, everyday things and take very small steps. I always had a beer in my hand, and now I don't. But I'm aware that I don't, and I feel awkward. So I put a Coke in my hand instead. It helps. So much of this is adjusting to 'new ideas.' I used to like to travel, but now I'm reluctant to go. It's a new idea not to drink on a plane! Or how can you have oysters without chardonnay? These are the kinds of things that can take me by surprise. But there's grief in letting go."

The therapist hears the natural building-block process of changing behavior and thinking underway, and may say so, supporting the process Irene has just described.

Deb Baxter (above) gives another example:

"The initial stage was awful. I was depressed for several months. It was the worst time in my life. Communication with Ron was sparse and difficult. My value system had to change, but it wasn't changing. During those days I focused everything on not drinking. It was hard for me to do anything that I used to do drinking, and by the end that was just about everything. I gave up Valium and drinking at the same time, and I had choices. Did I want to put myself in these situations without alcohol or tranquilizers? In the first year I said no to everything. I had to let the children see I couldn't do anything. I had to let them down. If I was going to be comfortable, I had to do my own thing."

The therapist hears that Deb was doing what she needed to do: focus on herself and say no. Yet Deb's family was upset. They didn't like the drinking, but what had happened to their mother now? They were tired of hearing about recovery and of hearing their mother say no. The therapist working with this family (1) acknowledges the pain of these experiences; (2) may explain why it is necessary at this point in time (though he or she must be careful not to defend the mother in a manner that causes guilt for unhappy family members); (3) assesses whether the spouse and children are getting help for themselves; (4) explores possible changes that might improve the family situation without compromising mother's attention to recovery; (5) and helps the family members cope with the reality and express their dissatisfaction.

Mick Lonergan sums up his shock on becoming abstinent:

"I had a fear of the unknown, and this was completely unknown. One day I said to myself, 'This lifestyle generated by alcohol has gotta change.' The early days were nothin' but fear, groping, and a black-and-white following of 12-step slogans and rules."

Many individuals recall that they feared the void without alcohol, an emptiness that would overwhelm them in sobriety. Alcohol filled the void and deepened it, but the idea, while they were still drinking, of relinquishing alcohol without a replacement was unimaginable. In Transition, people replace alcohol with a relentless focus on recovery: new actions and new substitutes for alcohol, such as AA meetings, friends, and for some the belief in "something greater," a "Higher Power," in AA terms.

The Coalcoholic in the Transition Stage

In the drinking phase of Transition the world of the coalcoholic grows increasingly narrower and more isolated as the individual becomes more occupied by the demands of the alcoholic system and the alcoholic. The partner intensifies his or her attempts to control the alcoholic and to rescue or just hold together the alcoholic family system that is heading toward collapse. Coalcoholics may or may not hit bottom before their alcoholic partners. If they go first, their surrender to reality—that they cannot control the alcoholic or hold the family together any longer—may sooner or later (or never) be a catalyst for the alcoholic to hit bottom too. Or it may work the other way. Len Irving, whom we met in Chapter 8, recalls the changes in the home and in his feelings as his denial crumbled:

"There was a period of surrender of about 2 months. I had been seeing a therapist for some time, certain that I was crazy. It was so stressful, I couldn't cope any longer. Life is a lot of bending and stretching, but this was a tearing of the fabric. My therapist kept telling me that Jane was alcoholic and I just couldn't see it. Those last two months, my therapist 'shook it into me' and it sunk in completely. It got to my bedrock. As I let this new reality in, things got worse and worse at home."

Pam Richardson (above) recalls that the turning points for her centered on her becoming more receptive to information as Matt's alcoholism began to permeate the family environment and system. This is a reversal of the shutting off and shutting down of denial. We also see a slower shift in direction from digging deeper into the underground morass of alcoholism to digging up and out of it. Pam remembers:

"My life was perfectly happy for years. Matt drank, but it didn't involve me and it didn't involve our family. I wasn't complaining. But in the last 3 years the family atmosphere was disrupted. He was failing his commitments and not showing up. I began to expect that our reliable routines would be disrupted. I got some Al-Anon literature and then a book about alcoholism and the family that laid it all out. I became receptive to seeing reality. As I learned more, I changed my behavior, and that pushed Matt. He was already worried, but now he started a process of seeking help. He didn't stop drinking and neither he nor I really began our separate recoveries until we hit a terrible crisis."

Alison Hunter remembers hitting bottom as she moved from "coping" to "action" when her alcoholic husband attempted suicide:

"I couldn't ignore it anymore—there was plenty of evidence. He was a danger to himself and me. I was scared. A friend referred me to an 'Interventionist' who was the first person who ever told me how sick I was. She was the bluntest person I'd ever met. She 'intervened' on me before him—how I'd deadened myself in order to function. I was so depressed and crying all the time. I saw that our life together was extremely fragile. I had to go from my usual authoritative, controlling mode to receiving help. The intervention was a 'ceremony of significance' for both of us. Our present situation would be very different if we hadn't gone through this together."

The abstinent side of Transition is often more difficult for coalcoholics than was trying to cope with active drinking, though all may feel grateful for recovery. Paula Simons describes her anxiety early on:

"In the beginning I was uptight. I was unstable with the new. I had no faith or trust. I would sneak around checking on him. Trust built slowly. Then, suddenly, I had a calm, peaceful feeling within."

People are often dramatically confronted with their fantasy that sobriety was supposed to mean "no more problems." Coalcoholics are often shocked at the depth and extent of their own denial: they have been as "addicted" to focusing on and controlling the alcoholic as that individual has been addicted to alcohol. The process of beginning recovery for the coalcoholic includes the following: challenging denial; accepting the identity of coalcoholic, or the role as a partner in an unhealthy drinking system; learning recovery behavior and thinking; and focusing on the self. The therapist monitors the process and helps the patient explore resistance.

Karen Graham was very angry about her husband's abstinence and the pain she felt:

"I was always taught to take care of disease, to be helpful and loving. Now, I was told not to be helpful, which was baffling to me. I was all caught up in drinking—the attitudes and behaviors of the whole system. There was a lot of confusion."

Recovery was a shock. Karen did not want to hear that her loving, kind actions were part of the family pathology of drinking. She was furious that she was identified as a "coalcoholic" and that her efforts to help her husband were not seen as valuable. It got worse. She was now identified as part of the problem, but Bill still got all the attention. Many coalcoholics told us that they felt heard and understood by professional treatment people until their alcoholic mates went into treatment and recovery. Then they felt abandoned and blamed for having any needs from their partners who were now so focused on recovery. Karen recalls:

"It's a dilemma for the codependent; you're part of a system, so when the alcoholic goes to treatment there's a void and feelings come out. All the attention was on Bill, but I needed attention too. Bill was in the recovery limelight, 'King Baby' as I saw it. All my bad traits, like jealousy, came out. It brings out the dark side.

I had no idea what I was 'letting go' of, so I didn't 'let go' of the negative and the destructive. The person who is not anesthetized with alcohol must deny it all or go insane. As my denial broke, I had to become more awake to the damage that was done."

Coalcoholics entering recovery are involved in the same major process of change as the alcoholic is. They are faced with the need to focus on themselves as opposed to the alcoholic or the couple. At this point, many coalcoholics simply do not grasp that they have a separate self to focus on. Thus, many resist, as Sherry Sussman illustrates:

"I was so angry with the therapists who told me to go to Al-Anon. It wasn't about me as far as I was concerned. All the kids had trouble too. They wouldn't see themselves as ACOAs.

"In this early time I 'endured.' I felt like Eric's sponsor or his mother. I was happy if he could control his impulses. And, I was arrogant; I thought Al-Anon was beneath me."

One of the most difficult realities that the coalcoholic must face is coalcoholism; that is, the partner of the alcoholic has been reactive to and therefore deeply involved in sustaining the alcoholic drinking system. Just what does this mean? Often, it is a devastating reality, only slowly acknowledged. Some coalcoholics have never seen themselves as part of the problem. In fact, they may have assumed the burden of full responsibility for the family, a role in which they (like Karen Graham) often see themselves as heroic. Underneath, though, the coalcoholic may have felt deeply to blame—for everything going wrong and nothing going right. The children often can't understand how the nonalcoholic parent could have gotten so out of control.

Sue Thompson recalls the move toward finding her own recovery:

"A big jump came in my Al-Anon recovery when Harvey stopped telling me to go to Al-Anon. First, Al-Anon was something for him. Then it became something for me. I was addicted to Harvey, and I had to recognize it. He was gone, and I was in agony. Harvey was my lifeline."

Recovery frequently represents loss as much as hope, and the unknown as much as any return to a "normal" that may have preceded alcoholism. Couples in which both partners begin a separate recovery process tell us that they don't go back to normal. This is something new.

The Children in the Transition Stage

As we look at children, it's time to say again that recovery is a good thing. We must emphasize this positive change, because so much of Transition is so hard and often quite negative for children as well as adults. It's important to remember that this shift in everything, this turning upside down and inside out, eventually passes. Otherwise, it may be hard to sustain positive feelings about abstinence. At this point, it often seems much worse than drinking. Kids can weather Transition well if they are protected, informed in age-appropriate terms, and reassured, all tasks for the therapist and the parents. Pam Richardson remembers:

"We were in an uproar—chaos. And this was after Matt went to treatment. The kids felt their whole world crumbled after he stopped drinking. Several weeks into treatment, we became an identified 'alcoholic family' and things started to get better. That identity gave us stability and a way of understanding what was happening. We began to make sense of all that we had hidden and denied during the drinking. The kids didn't like it at all—this was a nightmare—but it was reality and naming it helped us all over time."

Transition is characterized by massive change that affects children at every level. The move toward the end of drinking is often extremely traumatic. So is abstinence. There is just as much or more uncertainty, fear, and tension in the environment as the family members face the void of new abstinence without a healthy family structure to hold them. Children often feel more unsafe than they felt during the drinking because everything is now unknown and unpredictable. Many of the children in our research said they worried a lot about whether or when a parent was going to drink, or become angry or enraged in response to the anxieties of withdrawal and new abstinence. The environment feels unsafe for the first few months. Depending on the degree of security and protection provided by the parents, it may remain unsafe for much longer. Both parents may be absent and not paying attention to children. Violence may continue. For most families, it is still a context of chronic trauma, with the dark smoke of an impending "something bad" hanging over all. Some families may deny their worries, focusing instead on the relief of abstinence.

On the family systems level, children feel bewilderment and confusion because they do not understand what is happening. The parents are making changes, yet the changes are likely to bring more confusion and chaos than relief. Unfortunately, as we highlighted in Part I, there can be a sad paradox: when the drinking system collapses and both parents reach outside the family to recovery resources (which is exactly what they need to do), the children may feel, and actually may be, abandoned. Ironically, they may be more abandoned than they were during the drinking. And they may be more frightened if no one knows what is happening and no one is in charge of their care.

The child's experience with abstinence depends on circumstances during the drinking and the end of drinking and how parents are coping with Transition. Sometimes, as we saw earlier (in Chapter 8) with Betsy Jameson and her son Tim, the child is protected and insulated from active involvement in the trauma of drinking. One parent can label the alcoholism and face it directly to ensure the child's safety and the acknowledgment of reality. The move to abstinence may not be as cataclysmic as it will be for the child whose parents have denied any problem with alcohol until a severe crisis propels them toward the end and the family has been thoroughly traumatized by the process of hitting bottom and beginning abstinence. There is often a need for crisis intervention as parents have lost or abdicated sufficient caretaking in this time of intense trauma.

Sam Yarrow, whom we also last met in Chapter 8, told us that he spent the first 2 years of his parents' recovery alone in his room with his headphones on. He knew there would be something to eat in the house, but he didn't know what or when. He tried not to be upset or feel needy, because both his parents were working so hard on their recoveries.

We hear the painful loss of Sam's parents, along with his stoic role reversal, as he tries to be supportive of them.

As parents reach out for their own programs of abstinence, it is important that they, or substitutes, attend to parenting responsibilities inside the family. Kids generally need the structure of a healthy family system, which at this stage we know does not likely exist and thus can't be called upon. Instead, like their parents, they know the unhealthy systems dynamics that supported the drinking family. They may wish that their parents would drink again, or they may act up to draw the parent's attention to them.

Children need the same kind of support that their parents are receiving. This includes education about alcoholism that is appropriate to the child's age, and opportunities to share their own feelings about what has been and is happening. In many treatment centers, children's groups provide this support. Counselors can also help parents keep abreast of their children's needs as recovery begins. It is important that parents provide enough information about what is happening to calm a child's fears, but not so much that the child is frightened or called upon to solve the parents' problems. This is likely to be a tricky middle ground since the children often have been too intensely involved in the family's alcoholism.

As therapists, we must support the parents' abstinence and help them attend to their children. We do not support parents in further damaging their children by ignoring them or denying their needs. It does no one any good to continue to harm children with the rationale that it is necessary for the parent. As we've already noted, some parents took better care of their children when they stopped drinking and some felt terrible guilt about the continued damage their kids were suffering on behalf of the parents' recovery. We should acknowledge to the parents that this double focus is hard and work with them to restructure their daily schedule to allow the best mix of attention to themselves and their children. Accordingly, we recommend AA or Al-Anon meetings that provide childcare or residential treatment centers that include children. If these are not available, we suggest community alternatives, which are growing. We assess the parents' ability to be competent and to provide for their children's safety. When necessary, we recommend additional outside services and may alert authorities.

Confusion in role is problematic for all. Old roles don't fit anymore, but new ones aren't clear or even possible because the family is in such turmoil. The child "hero/ heroine" who used to feel and behave like a responsible parental figure may become intensely competitive with his or her parents who are now themselves at last learning to behave like responsible adults. Another child may act up in response to changes in the system and the threat of the unknown of abstinence. This child may react strongly to a parent's appropriate exertion of authority, experiencing new parental limits as demeaning and infantilizing. New family rules also may be enforced with rigidity and confusion since parents are not yet comfortable in this responsible role.

The emotional relationship between the parents is likely to be painful and strained for a long time into abstinence. The move toward hitting bottom may have included the threat of divorce or separation, frequent arguing, and all too often violence. As already noted, the parents need to separate emotionally during this early time to focus on their individual recoveries. Yet this necessary separation may be extremely anxiety provoking to a child who longs for stability and reassurances that all will be well. Unfortunately, no one yet knows what will happen. Children need to feel confidence that they are loved and will be protected and attended to even though the parents are so busy with their own recoveries. Children need to be protected so they can focus on themselves and proceed with their own development. But this is hard, as Trish tells us:

> "I was growing up with alcoholism, which was perfectly normal. Then came recovery. I remember feeling scared and baffled. How could I separate what was family dysfunction now and before from what was me, being 9 years old? All of us were going through our own stages, and it was very confusing."

Marcus Frasier, 18, whose alcoholic father, with 4 years of abstinence now, used to verbally rage and physically attack him, reflects back:

> "In the first 2 years, whenever he was gone, I was happy. When he was using booze and gone, I was happy. I didn't have to hide. When they would go to meetings, I wouldn't have to be afraid; I could be free to live. We still butt heads, but I stand up for myself."

His mother, who is also a recovering alcoholic, remembers what it was like for her as a mother:

> "It was more devastating for me after my first treatment because I went back out [she started drinking again]. Now I understood what I was doing to my children, and I was tormented. I was being abusive, inconsistent, and I wasn't going anywhere."

Marcus continues:

"It was harder when she started drinking again. We'd been in recovery—I'd gone to Alateen—and it wasn't me slipping. But being a child, I couldn't do anything. We no longer could be a family in recovery because she was drinking and everybody had stopped going to meetings. We had a 'family slip.' I stopped reading, no meetings. I went back into being awful.

"Then I knew this wasn't right. I knew they could be clean, healthy, and available. People's true personalities came out in recovery, so I knew what was possible. Before, when they were drinking, it was normal because we didn't know. It was normal for them to be unstable. They were even predictable. It was chaotic, but we knew what to do. Now, it was much worse. I'd had a taste of recovery and then I had it taken away. It was pretty devastating."

Relationships between siblings may also change. Intense ties that evolved in the absence of strong parental figures may be loosened as parents become more involved with the family. A child who was previously a substitute spouse may attempt to parent younger sibs who may rebel. Or sibs may become closer, forging bonds in the absence of their parents, who are now so focused on themselves, and/or because the environment is healthy enough for the sibs to do so.

Uncertainty and fear about their parents and the future well-being and even survival of the family may be expressed in depression, sleep disturbances, mood instability, and behavioral problems. Not infrequently, adolescents begin drinking and using drugs themselves. Trish Lowell describes it:

"I'm out of the program now. I lost my adolescence and my childhood. I had to become a parent. Now I have to go out and be irresponsible. I won't be able to go far from recovery because of my parents. I've got all the characteristics to be an alcoholic, but I hope I don't have to."

In some families, children are expected to assume the roles of children once abstinence begins. This straightening out of role may feel like a great loss to a child who has derived self-esteem from an unhealthy family role that is no longer needed. Any sense of having a special bond with one or both parents may be lost, with no nurturing or attention from the parent to replace it. Or children may have had a weak and mostly negative bond with drinking parents. They may be unaffected by the parents' move into recovery unless they do receive attention, which is likely to be simultaneously welcome, confusing, and not to be trusted—yet.

One of the main reasons Transition is so hard for children is the often drastic change in reality. What was denied before, the drinking, is now the acknowledged focus of everything. It is a shock to kids to have their parents change their view and explanations of reality so dramatically and quickly. This threatens the child's developing experience of self and challenges the child's confidence in his or her own perceptions, explanations, and feelings. Children who grew up with alcoholism as "normal," find new recovery very abnormal and often terrifying. As parents remain in various stages and states of denial themselves in this critical period, their view of reality is likely to be confused and confounded by the distortions of the drinking that continue side by side with the rapid shift to telling the truth in recovery. One ACOA told her family in the interview that they were in as much denial as before, only now it wasn't about the drinking. And Karen Graham told us above that her "dark side" came out with abstinence.

In another family, we observed that the mother, who had been in charge during the drinking, lost too much control of defining reality in abstinence. Her son said that the whole family contributes to writing the story of family recovery but Mom is the editor. She is still in charge of what can be known and said.

The outside educator can be enormously helpful to the receptive family. As Pam Richardson said above, becoming an "identified alcoholic family" calmed everybody down. It was general education about alcoholism and family dynamics that helped, providing structure and a map, rather than sorting through the family members' defenses at this early date.

Children may experience a parent's abstinence and the intense focus on recovery as a terrible intrusion into their own normal development, as Trish Lowell noted above. We found that, depending on many different family circumstances, preadolescent children are better able to join parents in the new process of family recovery, adjusting their views of their lives and reality to match the changing perceptions and beliefs of their parents. As kids get closer to adolescence, they feel more threatened by the sudden change in reality. They are approaching the beginnings of detachment and separation and may feel thwarted when the family loses its stability, even though abstinence is positive. Adolescents indicate that they are too close to growing up to change their entire view of themselves.

Education and tremendous support are essential. But people still feel the pain. Tim Jameson (Chapter 8) said he worries that his father, Roy, will drink. He's grown close to Roy in recovery but sadly anticipates the time when his father will relapse. It's happened before. Even though Tim's mother is always there and he's had the support of Alateen, he feels lonely and sad when Roy is off on a binge.

Well, is there anything good to report? Yes. Abstinence is good. But everybody needs help at this point and nothing is sure. Nobody can trust much of anything. It's important to know that this is normal and this is OK. No wonder it's so hard to survive the Transition stage and even build on this vulnerable, chaotic time without outside support.

The therapist assesses the degree to which each family member is attached to individual recovery and moving positively in the behavioral, cognitive, affective, and spiritual process. The therapist points out what is normal and wonders about people's adjustment and resistance. If all goes well, the recovery process takes over and the therapist stands ready to facilitate forward movement. Things do get better, as we'll soon see.

CHAPTER TEN

Early Recovery for Couples and Families

Early Recovery brings increasing calming, a steady ease into the ongoing growth process that was set in motion during Transition. In this chapter, we'll see how things improve, but we'll also examine changes that are not necessarily happy or positive or easy to cope with. What keeps people going? It's so much better than before, and the building process gives people hope. This is the ripple effect: the positives build on the positives, which brings a greater experience of safety, trust, and hope. Are there negatives? Yes, and they can sometimes be overwhelming. But the skills are in place to weather a lot of rough seas.

If we focus on the individuals—the alcoholic and the coalcoholic partner—we'll hear the process of steady, healthy growth in place. If we focus on the couple, we'll get a different picture. If all goes *well*, the couple focus will still not be primary. Many will ask: How can this be? Who's going to wait this long? Good questions. Unfortunately, in our view, a lot of couples don't wait. Marriages end. To weather this long period of change, it takes trust and a commitment to the process, which couples develop in several ways. They benefit from the positive building from their own individual experience. They've learned that awful, seemingly unresolvable conflicts can and do get better. Many problems look different from the vantage of longer recovery, and couples become better able to deal with issues. They have tools now which they can turn to quickly in difficult times. For many, these

218

include an established relationship with a sponsor who has likely had similar experiences, the 12-steps that serve as action directives, and perhaps a solid relationship with a therapist.

On a global level, the therapist continues to assess movement and the critical issues in all the domains, pinpointing sources of difficulty or arrest. The therapist maintains a watchfulness as monitor, coach, and perhaps active therapist in a problem-solving or uncovering process. Now is the time when intensive psychotherapy may be necessary or desirable in dealing with resistances, past or present, to continuing growth. Yet the matter of resistance is complicated. The therapist must always carefully assess whether resistance and defense are blocking recovery or facilitating it. In Transition, individuals and couples may exert great defense, in the service of maintaining new abstinence, by tabling in-depth exploration of anything. By Early Recovery, the purpose of defense may be less clear. The therapist should work slowly, step by step, to determine which issues or feelings need attention and which do not. Our caveat remains: the therapist is guided by a focus on loss of control and the maintenance of abstinence.

In a counseling setting, the therapist assesses recovery progress: Where are people in their programs of recovery? What stage are they at? What issues are coming to the fore? Are meetings in place and attachments to recovery secure? If not, why? The therapist knows that individual issues from the past will be coming into focus, particularly as people begin a step 4 (making "a searching and fearless moral inventory" of themselves; Alcoholics Anonymous, 1952, 1955). They may experience anxiety, depression and other compulsive problems—overspending or overeating, for example—that signal a need for in-depth exploration and express the uncertainties and pain that are rising to consciousness.

Many people seek more intensive individual psychotherapy to facilitate and support 12-step work. People may also benefit from couples therapy in which the therapist follows the same protocol: first charting the normal process of recovery for both partners, then looking for resistance to the normal flow and addressing blocks at environmental, systems, and individual levels. Arlene and Ted Boxer illustrate a couple in which the therapist exercised a combination of approaches: after assessing individual recovery programs and the couple relationship in recovery, the therapist takes a psychodynamic view, recognizing that unconscious factors are intruding into the natural process.

Arlene became seriously depressed when her alcoholic husband marked his third sobriety birthday. She had become vigilant and chronically tearful, and neither partner had any idea what was wrong. They sought couples therapy because of the rupture they felt in their strong recovery partnership. The therapist checked on program: Both identified themselves as in recovery, both maintained a regular schedule of meetings, and both had good relationships with sponsors. They felt they each had strong individual recoveries and a good couple bond. Yet the environment had become tense as both tried to push the reality of Arlene's depression out of awareness. The openness the two had established was gone; both were defended and had begun to fight. The therapist, in taking individual histories and learning that Arlene's father had died in a car accident shortly after her third birthday, quickly recommended individual therapy for her. She responded well, seeing that she had unconsciously been reacting to Ted's happy sobriety birthday with deep mourning—exactly what she had experienced following her father's death. With therapy, she could see that she had carried mixed feelings about Ted's AA birthday celebrations since year 1. She had unconsciously expected that her husband would die or that he would drink and she would lose him.

The therapist worked with the couple to stabilize their environment and system in recovery by keeping them focused together in the present. This helped Arlene separate her past experiences from her current relationship. She continued in individual therapy.

One partner may still be ahead of the other, a difference that may cause severe conflict or a growing distance. Individuals who each have a focus on the self report the greatest satisfaction as a couple in this stage: they are busy and are no longer looking to the partner for self-fulfillment. Of course, partners may still interpret this necessary emotional separation as evidence that the marriage is failing. Not so, or at least not automatically so. It's part of the normal process of recovery. Let's follow the family through the first few years.

OVERVIEW

In Early Recovery people are settling into new identities as an alcoholic and coalcoholic, and settling into abstinent behavior. They no longer feel helpless and frightened most of the time, and they may well be sharing their own experiences with others—as peers and even as sponsors. They are still very focused on alcohol, but with less intensity than during Transition. Individuals have passed the crises of hitting bottom and beginning abstinence and, if they have developed a reliance on external supports, they are settled into the new learning and practicing of recovery. The outside supports of AA and Al-Anon, which are becoming familiar and even routine, help people maintain abstinence behaviorally. This opens the way for cognitive construction and reconstruction of the individual's identity as an alcoholic or coalcoholic to proceed. Both thought and action may now have a broader focus than containing impulses to drink. For example, people may be able to listen longer and better in meetings and to go between meetings with less craving. People begin to experience a sense of safety and a trust that, if they "work the program," they can remain abstinent. That frees them from the intense vigilance of Transition, where they must focus on action constantly, substituting an abstinent behavior for the impulse to drink. Still, they are watchful and attentive to signs of danger or relapse, which is always a possibility.

Coalcoholics simultaneously learn what it means to be coalcoholic and how to maintain a focus on the self instead of an addictive focus on the alcoholic. They too are less dominated by impulse and anxiety about their partners, and thus they are better able to learn about themselves through listening to the experience of others and beginning their own recovery programs.

Early Recovery is primarily a period of intense education and support for new behaviors, as well as attention to the self and individual growth. Here we see the critical importance of a shared language, available when both partners are in recovery programs. As individuals shift from a predominant behavioral focus to the cognitive challenge of belief and the construction of a new narrative, the shared language enables them to maintain a bond together while the focus is still heavily on them as individuals. It is as if the focus on alcoholism and the language that describes it serve to hold partners together until they can turn their attention back to themselves as a couple. At the same time, the labeling, and the creation of individual stories builds a new couple foundation based on a shared reality, or at least a shared framework for making sense of the past. In these discussions, people can begin to experience holding both an "I" and a "we," that is, the "I" of the individual self and the "we" of the couple.

Many couples don't know how to talk with each other. One individual said that she and her husband had always communicated with their emotions and behavior. Now that they can talk, they are shocked to realize they don't know how. Some say they have little in common; and without shared experience and language, this is often true. It is especially difficult if one partner is developing a story of drinking and recovery that the other denies is true. Some will end their relationship at this point.

Early Recovery is almost always a rugged time for the couple. It has to be. They have the remembered relationship organized around drinking, with little or nothing yet to replace it. Many agree that they never had a healthy sense of self and they never had a healthy couple relationship, even before drinking. Their couple bond was formed around alcohol. In Early Recovery, they experience a vulnerability in the system because of their absence of history together without alcohol.

Some couples reclaim a healthy bond and relationship that they had prior to alcoholism. These are partners who came together, and thus have a history together, before alcohol. They may have had a positive, strong system and healthier selves, which were submerged by the defensive dominance of the alcoholic system they created. When the need for defense is removed, their healthier prealcoholic selves may begin to flourish. Often, the memory and history of the stronger bond holds these couples through hard times in Early Recovery. But for most couples recovery brings a vacuum.

The therapist takes a careful couple history as well as individual histories to help anticipate and understand the flow of recovery. The therapist helps the couple recall their strengths and suggests small steps they can take to begin a foundation for a new system, still accenting the centrality of individual recovery. The therapist may also remind the couple that they never had anything else but an alcoholic system, so it's no wonder they are having such a hard time now.

Couples will lead parallel lives until there is a stronger sense of oneself and separateness from the other. At this stage, the individual's needs take precedence and the system slowly becomes redefined and redeveloped as it follows the growth of the individuals.

Early Recovery is a long stage accented more by degrees of accumulated and evolutionary growth than the rapid, radical instability and change of Transition. Individuals remain active in the first few years of Early Recovery, with lots of attention to behavior and building each person's story, or drunkalogue. As denial and other defenses lift, the learning curve takes off. Individuals in AA and Al-Anon will begin to "work the steps" (Alcoholics Anonymous, 1952). This involves self-reflection and a beginning process of acknowledging reality in the past and the present. The work of therapy is to facilitate this expanding, foundation-building process and to challenge defenses that get in the way.

Later on in Early Recovery, from 3 to 5 years and even longer, there is stabilization, predictability, consistency, and confidence in recovery. Now, the process is less focused on behavioral change and much more directed toward increasing self-awareness and self-knowledge. This is almost always a mix of emotional pain, relief, and pleasure. Many of our couples told us clearly that the changes that were possible for them at 5 years of abstinence could not have occurred at 6 months or even 3 years. Change is a building, evolutionary process that unfolds and grows from within. It is not imposed, nor can it be acquired. As one individual told us, "It's an inside job."

It's sometimes hard to tell the difference between Early and Ongoing Recovery because growth and change never cease. In Early Recovery, the couple relationship remains second in line to the individual focus, though partners may be very involved with each other. Recall what Ron Baxter told us in Chapter 9: he and Deb committed themselves to recovery (as individuals), which is not the same as committing to each other (as a couple). In Ongoing Recovery, both partners can shift their attention to the couple with a healthy foundation of individual growth in place. As we'll see in Chapter 11, attending to the couple relationship does not mean that partners must give up attending to themselves or their individual recoveries. Yet this is exactly what many fear. If all goes well for the individual and the couple, the therapist maintains a supportive, holding role. If all does not go well, the therapist intervenes more actively.

Now is a particularly rough time for the Type II couple. The partner who is engaged in recovery wants to embrace self-exploration enthusiastically. The other partner continues to resist this attachment to recovery for him- or herself and perhaps for the partner too. There is often a strong crosscurrent: the growth of one is a threat to the other. The therapist points this out repeatedly and wonders what keeps them in this unequal, unresolved status quo. For example, the nonengaged partner may remain just as frightened of letting go of the symbiotic drinking system as the alcoholic was afraid of giving up alcohol. Remember Maggie Turner in Chapter 3: she just could not understand what a focus on herself meant.

Sometimes resentment and anger from the drinking years cannot be dealt with in depth yet—but also can't just be bypassed. The damage of drinking simply looms too large. Many couples do not tackle the past in an in-depth way until many years into recovery.

It is important that the therapist follow the path of the couple and avoid second-guessing (say, by deciding that with 3 years of abstinence it's time for the couple to open up the past). If the therapist hears that the past is in the way and is contributing to arrested growth or other problems in recovery, then the therapist says so. The therapist assesses the stability of abstinence and the threat of relapse. Couples may stay stuck for a long time because they fear a relapse or the end of the relationship if they open up the problems. Yet they also fear a relapse or the end of the relationship if they don't. These couples may need more intensive psychotherapy.

Before we go to the domains, let's hear from a couple with 2 years, 9 months of abstinence. Well into Early Recovery, Henry and Iris Cameron contrast their long process of Transition, including relapse and a full return to drinking, with the experience of solidity and commitment to recovery that they both have now:

HENRY: A number of years ago, I went off to treatment without much struggle. I bought the whole thing and became a student of alcoholism. I viewed myself as "fixed—this was in the past." I thought everyone should go through the group experience of treatment. I had no fear of slipping because I was determined. One night I was happy and I took a drink. Just like that. Never thought a minute about it. From then on, I rejected AA. I thought, "these are not my people." I didn't get it.

Henry illustrates his failure to hit bottom and recognize his powerlessness and loss of control. By viewing himself as fixed and relegating drinking to the past, he closed off the process of new growth. In essence, he strengthened his will and his belief in his ability to control himself, so he could not be open to learn from others. He was simply going through the motions.

Henry further illustrates his inflation of ego and the buildup of defense when he says, "I bought the whole thing." The therapist knows that this kind of "conversion" leads to a false attachment and an abdication of self to the control of another, such as occurs in some cults. With alcoholism, surrender leads to an acceptance of loss of control and an assumption of responsibility for the self, which is exactly the opposite. In 12-step programs, being responsible involves asking for help and then taking the necessary steps to be abstinent and accountable. There is much confusion about these paradoxes. Therapists, just like their patients in recovery, should remain wary of easy, quick "success."

A therapist working with Henry during this time might have questioned the ease and speed with which he got "fixed." The therapist could have asked him if he believed he had lost control and, if so, was that belief guiding him? If not, what happened? Why had he reinstated his belief in control? The therapist could directly express his concern that Henry had built up his defenses and was not open to learning.

HENRY: (*continuing*) I crept back to drinking, thinking I could turn it off and on. Now that it had been recognized as a problem by me and everyone else, it had to be a secret. I couldn't drink in public, so I'd wait to get home to have a drink. It was an exciting way to live.

IRIS: I was aware of what was happening, and I knew when he was drinking, but I couldn't confront it.

HENRY: I was full of self-deception. I call that first treatment my "designer program": I took a little of this and a little of that. When you've got alcohol in your system, you're not thinking you've got alcohol in your system.

Henry describes the dynamics of self-deception, based on a belief in the power of self. He had to invoke more defenses—greater secrecy and distortion—to maintain his illusion of control. He thought he could turn his drinking on and off and convinced himself that that was what he was doing. Henry here illustrates the "grandiose self," a part of him that is propped up by alcohol but not consciously aware of the false inflation.

IRIS: I was amazed that recovery had broken down just at a time we were putting our lives together. We had a one-way conversation: he listened while I told him to "shape the fuck up." I was shocked at what I'd gotten myself into. This was a guy who was not in control and had no insight. He had to play it all out, but I had no idea what "playing it out" would mean.

Henry: Her confrontation was hard, but it didn't solve my addiction. I just had to be more careful. I began to sneak drinks from a flask in the drawer, under the seat in the car, or I'd pour it into a pop-top can. I went "under cover."

Iris: Henry became suicidal, and I arranged for an intervention. His threat of suicide forced me from coping, which is what I'd been doing for years, into action.

Henry: The intervention made me furious. I was angry and walked out. Forty-five seconds later I walked back in and said, "You got me." It was the best thing that ever happened. I knew they were right, and I stopped pretending that things were OK. They were doing the loving thing and I'd better listen.

Iris: I was going to Al-Anon now and counseling. We had to give up intellectual control and let the spiritual side of our lives control us. We became devoted to the recovery process. We went to separate meetings and did it together. We feel like a great unfolding is occurring between us.

Henry: Before I viewed my life as merit badges. The more badges you collect, the better Scout you are. My résumé was loaded with badges. This is different. I'm in it for the duration. This is a process, not an accomplishment.

As Henry describes his pursuit of merit badges, the therapist thinks of him "going through the motions." He sees that Henry reflects one of our core assumptions: becoming abstinent can be an event; recovery is a process.

The interviewer asks Henry and Iris if they saw stages in the process of recovery:

Henry: My self-esteem returned right away because I was doing something positive and, at about 9 months, I wasn't lonely anymore. I began to understand what serenity really means. Before it meant being busy, occupied. Now, it was just being. This serenity has flooded my life.

I have also learned tools that work in all my life. Recently I met with my new sponsor and I still tried to control the meeting by setting the agenda. My sponsor said, "Let's do the first three steps," which are all about giving up control to a Higher Power. The meeting went just fine.

Henry had an ongoing struggle with relinquishing control, which is a core issue for most people. His sponsor gently pointed it out, which Henry could accept. A therapist might do the same thing, noting how hard it is to accept loss of control as a guiding principle that affects everything.

IRIS: The first year I was weeping. We had to decide whether to stay in the marriage or not. I was suffering from the amount of rage I was taking in from him, and he would say his rage had nothing to do with me. But I was getting it. I told him, "Each of us has our own part of the meadow. You're burning yours down, and it's crossing over into mine."

After the first year it was like being lifted up. As a couple, we converted from "We have to do this" to "This is our work." It began to take over our new life. Now it feels like we're living a life permeated by spirituality. The recovery process is an adventure, being retrained for life.

The therapist hears the report of the giving up of control, the surrender, with a corresponding shift in their attitudes about how this change would take place. They moved from the frame of needing to be in charge of change to the frame of an acceptance of process, a process that would hold and shape them.

IRIS: I had a new sense of self and began to flower. I'm more direct and able to confront difficult issues more kindly in my work and with Henry. Recovery is finding the humility to get out of denial and finding the humility to get out of self-sufficiency.

Let's go now to the domains.

THE ENVIRONMENT

In Early Recovery, change is usually slower and less radical, although family crises may punctuate the steady process of change and growth. The overall context of the environment will feel calmer and safer, unless other family members have replaced the alcoholic and the alcoholism as the focus of crisis. It is not unusual for someone in the family to rush in, without conscious awareness, to fill the void created by abstinence with out-of-control behavior or new problems, such as illness, that require attention. Many alcoholic families are used to living in a chaotic, intensely emotional environment, which comes to feel normal. They still need external stimulation to feel anything, so extended abstinence may cause a new kind of anxiety, tension, and confusion. The quiet and the focus on individuals may feel very threatening. The therapist explains this expected state of affairs.

The trauma of recovery (i.e., adjusting to the sudden change brought by abstinence and the collapse of the drinking family system) continues. The uncertainty of the new adds to the anxiety. Tanya Hoffman (in Chapter 9), who stopped drinking and started to attend AA at the same time as her husband, Steve, recalls the chaos of the first few years:

> "Steve was on a pink cloud. He loved it. I hated it. I was jealous and possessive. Steve was so self-obsessed, he could care less what I was doing. I brought people home, and he brought people home. It was so upsetting for our two young kids. We argued—'dueling programs' we called it. We didn't settle down for a long time."

A therapist working with Steve and Tanya early on might have intervened directly to protect their children. The therapist might also have functioned as a referee and coach, helping them find neutral ground so they could work together in support of their individual programs and their kids.

Other families move out of chaos sooner. Abstinence takes hold more firmly, and parents grow increasingly secure in new behaviors and recovery routines. Mandy Wilkins describes it:

> "It's been a gradual settling in to routine. It's calmer, less jarring now. We started talking to each other at about 8 months, and somewhere about the same time it became easier to poke fun without taking offense."

These beginning positive, stable changes allow for some hope and even excitement, as Tanya and Steve's son Freddie recalls:

> "I hated it all. I hate coming here today. But it's a lot better. Both of them are fun, and I'm not embarrassed now. I like them; it's awesome."

Another family describes this period of new learning and change:

"We went from chaos to smooth. We can feel it, and we can see the change in everyone. At first, it was just a big blur."

In Early Recovery family members may have a difficult time interacting. They may have no idea how to approach each other and they fear making mistakes that could lead to feeling out of control. Everything feels unknown and unfamiliar. Jane Irving (whom we met in Chapters 8 and 9) tells us that being able to sit in the same room without a fight felt like a major victory. She also accents the unpredictability of it all:

"Family life centered on reacting to each other's craziness and comings and goings. It was all pretty chaotic. Len and I just kept taking it a step at a time, but the kids were saying, 'Where's supper?' It didn't quiet down for several years even though we were all pretty happy and loved recovery."

Children may feel frightened of the changes. They may not understand why their parents are away so much, and they may continue to feel abandoned. If uncertainty and unpredictability continue to characterize the environment, children may be traumatized by the vacuum—the absence of parents who could offer necessary support through this disruptive but potentially positive time of growth. Again, as we saw in Transition, the experience is mixed for most kids: they welcome sober parents and now have a history of solid recovery experiences with them; but they still fear the changes, particularly if parents remain less available than they were during drinking.

The therapist should assess the environment, first monitoring for safety and protection of children. Is this an environment in which kids can safely grow even if it is still uncertain and chaotic?

THE SYSTEM

In the beginning of Early Recovery new routines give a rudimentary start to family operation. The agreement to go outside the family to AA and Al-Anon, therapy, or other sources of support enables individuals to focus on themselves and to resist pressure to reinstate the old drinking system with its promise of familiarity. In fact, the inclusion of external supports becomes an interim system that allows the family to remain intact without a new internal structure to hold it. Recovery supports operate like extended family who have come for a long stay. The "presence" of AA and Al-Anon sponsors and friends automatically interferes with the old family system. Recall the couple in Chapter 9 who didn't make any decisions or even talk with each other during their first year without calling their sponsors. Some families look back and see these helpful outsiders as a saving grace—"We would never have survived as a marriage or a family without our sponsors"—while others remember the intrusion, the loss of the old family structure, and even the loss of the drinking system. Anxiety dominates for them. Holly Davis, whose mother has been sober for 8 years, recalls her annoyance at AA and her mother's sponsor:

> "I felt displaced as the most important person in my mother's life, though the role was not a healthy one. Even so, I resented her AA sponsor. She'd show up all the time and want to talk with us about family alcoholism. We weren't thrilled."

If all goes well during this time, the foundations for a new, healthy system are being laid by the focus on individual change. New rules, roles, and routines consistent with recovery provide the building blocks of a new, healthy family structure. In many families, new rituals related to recovery are also in place. Celebrations of abstinent birthdays are an example. By the time Early Recovery is fully stabilized, new systems growth is well underway.

The therapist assesses the degree of chaos and difficulty in building a new system throughout Early Recovery. The ease or struggle of this reconstruction often depends on whether and how family members are accepting and adjusting to the new reality and routines. The therapist monitors change with a systems perspective in mind: Does everybody accept the reality of alcoholism? Do all members identify as an "alcoholic family"? How relieved are they about abstinence, compared to their anger over the disruption? Some families will be dealing with one crisis after another for several years. Others will quiet down sooner, with an easier focus on "working the program." During this stage we see big differences between families depending on whether one or both partners identify as being in recovery and whether they reach outside the family for supports. This may be the most important factor contributing to stability and ease of change in these first few years.

The Taylors, Jill and Peter, have demonstrated no systems change at all after several years of abstinence. They tell us they did not want their lives to be organized around alcohol. He has attended AA, but she has not attended any recovery program. Both see his continuing depression as their major couples issue.

The therapist's assessment is that both partners have organized their lives around coping with Peter's depression in the same way they had ordered their lives around alcohol. There has been no systems collapse and not much individual development. Worry about his depression has kept them bound in a symbiotic state.

The therapist might make these observations to Jill and Peter, offer suggestions to interrupt the system, and explore their resistance. Why has Jill never sought help? Why has she never attended Al-Anon? What would it mean and what would it be like if she focused on herself? What would it be like not to worry about Peter and not to feel responsible for curing his depression? What would it be like for Peter not to have Jill paying such close attention to him?

The therapist next assesses the length of time Peter has in abstinence and charts a good recovery program, which is in place. Peter attends meetings regularly and maintains contact with his sponsor. He berates himself constantly for not working a good enough program.

The therapist asks what is wrong with his program and hears that the more Peter deepens his work with the steps, the more depressed he gets, which Peter then sees as his failure. If he is working the steps, he should feel better. But working the steps brings into consciousness memories and feelings of Peter's childhood with two alcoholic parents. The therapist sees that Peter's movement in recovery has been arrested because of this past trauma and conflicts related to it. Peter feels guilty that he has survived drinking and is in recovery when his parents both died of alcoholism. He has also felt a loss of attachment to them since he stopped drinking. As Peter has become depressed, with progress in recovery, Jill has eased back into her coalcoholic position, re-creating the same enmeshed, symbiotic system they had during drinking. Their system is dry, but with an unhealthy structure.

Pam and Matt Richardson, whom we met in Chapter 9 and who entered recovery through a treatment center and then AA and Al-Anon, accented the importance of relying on outsiders:

"We got immediate feedback and a lot of learning about how normal families work from couples who had been sober longer. Before, we never discussed anything and now we do."

Pam and Matt illustrate the importance of having mentors, couples who have been in the recovery process longer who pass on their experiences. Beginning change is accomplished through imitation and modeling, learning that is not possible in a vacuum.

Partners usually experience a marked decrease in impulsive behavior—besides recovery behaviors, that is—and a new ability to tolerate anxiety. But neither of these changes applies very much to the couple relationship or to the workings of the family system. Partners are still likely to feel anxious and threatened about any and all family matters. Again, this anxiety may be lessened if they share the new language and experience of recovery.

Early Recovery is hard because new roles and rules are not yet well developed. Who does what is often a huge problem because who did what before was so unhealthy. Should the partner still make a doctor's appointment for the alcoholic? Should either partner clean the children's rooms? Should the coalcoholic stay home from a meeting to be with the children so that the alcoholic can go or vice versa? These decisions are the constant unknowns of early recovery, and they can be very difficult.

In drinking, some of what family members called "caring" behavior was, in fact, defensive, designed to protect and sustain the pathological system. As Karen Graham said in Chapter 9, she had long thought, at a conscious level, that assuming responsibility for her husband, which included hiding the realities and consequences of his drinking, was being caring and loving. People who are locked into maintaining unhealthy attachments are baffled that their behavior and motivations, which they see as caring, can contribute to and cause so many problems.

In Early Recovery, people assume responsibility for themselves. Much of the individual and couples work involves sorting out who is responsible for what. This is incredibly difficult. Most people have no idea yet what an equal relationship, based on individual autonomy, is. Both partners likely hold a schema that relationship involves the loss of self. One woman said:

"I have no idea how to be married without thinking about him first. So, that causes a huge problem: I don't know how to be in recovery, put myself first, and be married at the same time."

When the couple has no idea about how to set healthy boundaries, the therapist should work concretely on very small tasks. It is important to be specific in helping the couple determine when an action is supportive of individual recoveries and when it is not. On one occasion a husband decided that changing his schedule for his wife's convenience was a good thing, while on another occasion he determined not to make the same change because it would not be supportive of his recovery at that time.

Helping the couple learn how to make these "gray" distinctions is a valuable part of the road back together toward a healthy system. Much of mature relationship is not cut and dried, all or none. Yet holding ambiguity, or a "both–and" mentality, can be threatening early in recovery. A groundwork of problem solving and compromise that does not harm either partner will help the couple learn to maintain both an "I" perspective (on each of the individuals in separate recoveries) and a "we" perspective (on the couple) later.

Family members may feel resentment that the alcoholic wants to be involved in the family after being absent and disengaged for so long—or vice versa. The Robinson family resisted joining Dad in recovery for some time. They weren't in any hurry to welcome him back to the family, and, according to Alan, the father, they felt he was pushing too hard:

> "I was determined to assert myself back into the family. If they didn't like it, too bad. If it took yelling, then we'd do yelling. It didn't go over too well."

A partner may sabotage the efforts of the other to assume parental responsibility, or he or she may remain angry that the alcoholic is as unavailable as ever, having traded alcohol for AA. So what's different for the family, they may say? The drinker got all the attention before and now it's the same thing. Everything evolves around the alcoholic.

Feelings about "what it was like" now begin to emerge. Family members may be feeling, for the first time, the intensity of their anger toward the alcoholic and the coalcoholic. Their fantasy that sobriety will solve all the family's problems is not materializing, which may make family members doubt or question their abilities or even their commitment to maintain recovery. If the family has successfully shifted its focus off of the system onto the individuals within it, early recovery should be a time-out from major family reorganization beyond what is necessary to maintain recovery and the basics of family life.

Even relatively easy negotiation and decision making may be quite difficult because the couple may still be too polarized.

While we are saying it is not easy and many people are upset, there is also as much or more that is positive going on. Of our families who could say how hard it had been, most wouldn't change a thing. Certainly, they valued abstinence at any cost. For some, Early Recovery was all positive.

Typically, these were Type I families in which both partners identified in recovery. Some of these could be called "pink cloud" couples: they loved everything and simply denied any difficulties. Others were much more realistic but always framed their experiences from a positive slant. Yes, they had problems, but this was reality. Life is not easy. They were grateful for abstinence and the opportunity to grow, painful as that might be.

Usually, families who were in Early Recovery told us how good it was or how awful, and families who were looking back from 8 or 10 years of abstinence or longer could say more about both the good and the bad. It's simply easier to see clearly when looking back. It's also easier to acknowledge difficulties after surviving them.

In working with families in Early Recovery who can only think in sweeping good or bad terms, the therapist ought to listen for details. He or she may see and hear more difficult issues waiting to be dealt with after a solid behavioral and cognitive recovery program is in place. Or these same issues are causing relapse. When does a therapist raise a flag?

Back to our core assumptions: Is the construction process of recovery in place? Is it guided by a belief in loss of control and a commitment to abstinence? If people say that recovery is good, the therapist wonders how and why? What is good? Is the family's assessment true or is it covering problems, a pink cloud of denial heading toward relapse? If people say recovery is bad, the therapist wonders how and why? Are there ways for the therapist to help? Is there a systems block?

To learn about family systems problems and changes, we ask directly about communication, roles, and rules. One family, the Russells, Glen and Helen, with 29 months of recovery, and three grown children, all agree that big changes in communication have taken place very quickly. As Dirk, the oldest son, puts it, "We are naming things we used to hope would go away. We are less defensive, and more loving instead of angry and abusive." Susan, his sister, nods in agreement but adds, "Everything isn't quite so rosy. There's a lot that still can't be talked about." Other family members tell us in response that Susan is "always challenging about something." This discussion reveals a lot of family tension that they did not tell us about directly.

In a counseling setting, the therapist might pursue this comment, asking the family what kinds of things Susan was concerned about and asking Susan if she could say, and wanted to say, what wasn't being discussed. Or, instead of asking directly, the therapist might first comment on the tension in the room and note that Susan seemed to hold the role of family challenger. Staying at a systems, process level, the therapist might then ask family members how Susan got this role, and what purpose it served. They might more easily talk about the process than the content at this point. We might imagine, for example, that Dirk continues to drink, which, according to tacit family rules, no one can mention.

We also ask all our research families how decision making has changed. Most instantly recognize a difference. This is not something that couples have to stop and think about. They know they've changed and often can clearly state how. Yet most had never thought much about it till we asked. Glen Russell says, "Before it was all Helen, and I was along for the ride. I'm more assertive now. We discuss any major decisions." When we ask if they fight, Helen answers, "No, I clam up and walk away." Couples frequently remain frightened of anger and of sexuality throughout Early Recovery.

Why? The reasons can be complicated. On a concrete level, people fear that any change, including the potential for intimacy, may threaten abstinence. Feelings and the expression of anger and sexuality can involve loss of control, which stimulates anxiety, which stimulates a fear of drinking and/or a craving for alcohol. Alcoholics in recovery frequently report that they feel hung over after an emotional experience or that they have had a drinking dream following a fight with a partner. Unconsciously, people equate the release of emotion with being out of control, which they associate with drinking (Brown, 1985). These unconscious links last for years into recovery (or forever), though people become able to recognize them consciously. Understanding this fear of loss of control is essential for therapists and families. All change, regardless of how desirable, will likely feel threatening because the unknown carries a threat of loss of control.

Several parents have described a change in family structure when they declared the family to be a sober home. People could not enter if they had been drinking and no drinking or drug use would occur inside the home. This rule demonstrated parental authority in decision making and an agreement between parents about the primacy and organizing role of recovery. This rule, and others like it, strengthened the safety of the home and often set in motion a flow of positive change. The Russell children tell us they now love to visit their parents in the family's vacation home: "It's safe, it's fun, and we love to talk with Dad now."

For some families, new rules are like an alarm, setting off a rebellion. No one welcomes this sudden change and exercise of authority.

THE COUPLE IN THE EARLY RECOVERY STAGE

"You'd think things would be better by now." And they often are. But they aren't solved. In fact, the process of new couple development is just underway and it's often full of trial and error, starts and stops, and uncertainty about the future or whether there is any future. If you're a couple in Early Recovery, it sure helps to know "This is normal and this gets better."

As we've stated, during active alcoholism the needs of the individual are sacrificed to those of the drinking system. Now, the focus is on the individuals. Type I couples may settle into stable, parallel recovery growth. Type II couples have more trouble. Jenny Eaton, with 4 years of abstinence, tells us she was active in a recovery group, AA, and therapy during her first year. Her husband, Jake, was supportive of her but did not see that he had any problems or any need to pay attention to himself. Jenny says:

> "We coexisted during that year, but I could feel the gap between us widening. At 1 year I gave him an ultimatum. He needed to get some help for himself or we wouldn't make it. He did. For the next few years we still coexisted, but we were both moving and opening up to each other about ourselves. Our individual work was the new ground on which we could start talking. We never fought much before, and we don't now. We had sexual differences and problems before, and we still have the same issues. But we have started talking about it all. We are able to see our relation-

ship as mixed—positive and negative—which is very good. Before, it was all black and white; all good or all bad. We've changed our communicating and the way we make decisions. I guess I'd say it's all about talking. We talk and we never talked before. And we're able to tolerate not having answers; we can talk without always coming to a conclusion."

The Robinsons, Alan and Sherry, offer another example. They illustrate the tremendous growth and easing of barriers between them, along with a tolerance for staying in the process without answers. Alan tells us they were beginning now, at 3 years of abstinence, to see the outline of a new couple relationship. It was like a dim light on the horizon. Alan says he wasn't sure he still loved his wife at first. He was caught up in recovery, but she wasn't coming along. Sherry adds:

"I couldn't stop focusing on him. I just wanted to be supportive. I tried not to cause problems, and I avoided controversy. I felt so positive seeing him feel better. But it was hard for me not knowing about him. He wasn't telling me everything anymore, and I felt such loss. I really lost a part of him, and that part grew bigger. He had an entirely new life which was thrilling to him, but I wasn't a part of it. I tried to go to Al-Anon, but I couldn't do it."

A therapist working with Sherry and Alan during this early period would certainly have challenged Sherry's continuing focus on Alan and continued to recommend Al-Anon, perhaps gently and with humor, even though she refused to attend. The therapist would also have continued to question and explore her resistance. But Alan and Sherry were not in therapy. They had settled into a comfortable abstinence in which Alan was growing in recovery but Sherry wasn't. Alan continues:

"During this time, we saw all the differences between us we'd never been able to recognize. You do have to stop and see if there's enough to keep going, but a while back I began to think we don't look so bad."

Since the alcoholic used to focus on drinking and the coalcoholic used to focus on the drinker, the redirection of attention onto the self can be a significant challenge. As people are able to hold the focus on individual recovery and to take responsibility for themselves, they are better able to resist the pull to reengage in the hostile, blaming couple dynamic that most likely characterized their relationship during the drinking.

Some couples were disengaged during the drinking and find that little has changed in recovery. They may do well together during this time of individual focus and great emotional distance. Later, they may have more trouble as they become ready for intimacy and recognize the gulf between them and the absence of any history of closeness. The couple still doesn't have a new system, although they are well on the way with the foundation of their healthy individual recoveries. This is a key axiom: individuals cannot start out unhealthy and count on the partner or the couple relationship itself to fill a hole or heal them. That's an individual job.

Some partners benefit greatly from couple therapy that facilitates communication and dialogue without sacrificing autonomy and individual programs of recovery. Joanne Fulton told us that couple therapy helped her immensely during the first few years because Brian, her husband, grew almost completely silent when he stopped drinking. They had had a good relationship before, and now it felt awful. Brian would talk in the therapy, but he couldn't talk with her outside. She told us that she missed alcohol and she missed his drinking. She knew he was depressed, but she felt helpless to do anything about it. Joanne said it was 5 years before Brian started talking again.

A couple whom we have already met in Chapters 8 and 9, Jane and Len Irving, laughed and sighed ruefully as they talked about the long hard road of Early Recovery. They considered separating several times in the first few years because of the terrible tension between them. They didn't know how to be a couple after almost 30 years of marriage, and they thought they should call it quits. Before making the decision to end the marriage, they rented an apartment several hours away that was to be their symbol of separation *and* a free zone for them as a couple. Each could go alone to this apartment, and when they went together they agreed that it would represent positive recovery. At this pied-à-terre they would not try to solve couple issues, argue, or even discuss problems between them. This place was to provide a positive "time-out." Both said it offered them a neutral ground where they could "separate" without actually separating or ending their marriage, and they found a niche of closeness and trust in this declared "recovery" space that was impossible for them to find at home. At first it seemed like magic, but soon they realized it gave them a feeling of safety similar to what each felt in their 12-step programs. When they talked with us, they had 5 years of recovery. Len said their relationship had changed dramatically:

> "We used to try to talk about a problem, and we'd find ourselves spiraling into fighting. It was like an undertow. We couldn't stop the process from escalating, and we'd always end up raging and accusing. Now we can each pace ourselves and know when we need to stop, when we can't solve something, and when we are starting to roll back into that angry, defensive mode. Now, because we've done it and we've been successful, we can leave all kinds of problems unresolved because we know we'll come back to them—or they'll solve themselves, which is still a surprise. It's funny and embarrassing when we can't remember what we were fighting about just a day or two ago. There's a history and a foundation between us now that carries us so we can avoid going into that bad spiral of out-of-control anger."

Some couples settle into a stable recovery pattern quickly. Others struggle a long time. Cal and Jean Girard, sober for 7 years, had a long hard struggle as Jean recalls:

> "Early recovery was much worse than drinking. Cal would be on these 'dry drunks' where he'd argue about everything. He was 'in your face' with me and anyone who'd try to tell him anything. He thought he knew it all. Since he wasn't drinking, we'd have to deal with this constantly. He decided he was going to be a 'good homeowner.' Well, that meant that he needed, right now, this minute, a fancy lawn mower. He was out of control with the yard. Then he'd burn out, just like at the end of a binge, and that would be it. Then it would be something else. We separated after a year and stayed separate for a year. I would have left sooner if I'd had more Al-Anon."

Many couples survive Early Recovery. Many don't. It's overwhelmingly clear to us that reliance on outside supports and the ability to focus on the self are key elements for the survival of the couple. But it takes a lot more. Individual recovery is the cornerstone.

INDIVIDUAL DEVELOPMENT

The primary task of Early Recovery for each individual is to focus on alcohol and begin to integrate oneself into the environment of home and work as a recovering person. Optimally, each parent is building a new identity as a recovering alcoholic or a recovering coalcoholic. Early Recovery is marked by a decrease in impulses to drink or to focus on the alcoholic, a stabilization of behaviors, and an increased ability to tolerate anxiety.

For people in our research who belonged to AA and Al-Anon, and for those who did not but participated in therapy or some other avenue of self-exploration, Early Recovery is a time of new learning—about each person's vulnerabilities and how to take care of the self. For example, coalcoholics are learning how they lose themselves in relationships along with alternative behaviors and ways of thinking that will help them remain self-focused. Alcoholics are practicing and solidifying recovery behaviors and thinking. Both partners are watchful about signs and symptoms of potential relapse.

There is also a strengthening in basic identity as an alcoholic or coalcoholic through identification and new language, and a strengthening of the belief in loss of control. For those working the 12-step program, self-exploration deepens and broadens. It is often a time of awe and excitement about self-discovery.

Individuals are developing a sense of predictability and beginning to feel some stability within themselves. But confusion, disorientation, and depression are also common at this time of significant, steady change.

The Alcoholic in the Early Recovery Stage

Early Recovery is a continuation of all the radical changes and new learning of Transition, but it is less acute, less frightening, and less crisis dominated—at least for the most part. The need for substituting a recovery action in place of taking a drink is still paramount but usually not so urgent. Besides replacing the act of drinking, the new action counters a sense of void that comes normally with the removal of alcohol. New actions are also helpful in forestalling depression over the loss of alcohol, a common experience for most people early on. Action helps people cope, and action is the foundation for new learning. In a crunch, it is recovery actions that help people maintain abstinence.

In the Drinking stage there is no separation of thought and action; behaviors follow the conscious and unconscious desire to drink. In Transition, or early abstinence, thought and action may be distinct and yet connected. The individual experiences a desire to drink and must have a new behavioral alternative on which to act immediately. But by Early Recovery people also insert a new step between the impulse and the behavior, that is, the cognitive reminder "I am an alcoholic." AA supports people in learning to think before acting impulsively by using slogans such as "Fake it till you make it," "Old behavior = reaction, New behavior = action," and "Action rather than insight." Deb Baxter, whom we met in Chapters 8 and 9, recalls:

> "In the beginning, I focused on not drinking. All my decisions for a long time were based on not doing things that I had always done before in drinking situations. It was a conscious 'unhooking' of drinking from everything in my life. It's still important to me. I get anxious and careful every time I go through something for the first time that I used to do drinking."

Some people experience a honeymoon period, which we've already referred to as a "pink cloud," characterized by pleasure, elation, high self-esteem, and a denial of all other problems. Alan Robinson (above) called this time his "puberty," a time of awakening. This honeymoon period can be quite helpful, as it allows individuals to focus on being alcoholic, giving them an emotional "breather" from the difficulties of making changes while they are learning new behaviors and adjusting to the meanings of the identity "alcoholic."

Other people are not so lucky. They may experience much more loss, depression, and mourning, right from the onset of abstinence. Clinical experience suggests that women are more likely to miss the honeymoon period and more likely to struggle with depression early on (Brown, 1977; Kaufman, 1994). However, depression is a normal part of recovery for both men and women. Just when it hits, for how long, and how severe it is can differ significantly from case to case. It is important for the therapist (or assessor) to watch for depression and other emotional problems, such as anxiety, suicidal wishes or thoughts, sleep problems, fear, and/or helplessness, and to recommend professional help if necessary. This is an ongoing part of assessment.

Bart Harris, with 4 years of abstinence, talks mostly about his difficult emotional struggle:

"I don't know if I hit bottom with alcohol. I knew I was alcoholic. But after I stopped drinking I was really devastated with a terrible depression. It's been hard the whole way. I have a lot of anxiety and I've always had trouble sleeping."

We're back to emphasizing the importance of outside supports. Bart relied almost totally on Martha, his wife, for help. Both came to believe that he might commit suicide without her presence and attention. With this thinking, they created a dependence on each other similar to what they had when he was drinking. He maintained abstinence and was involved in AA, but he struggled because he could not establish a focus on himself. As Bart and Martha explained, his depression became the central focus of both of their lives in recovery.

One of the hardest realities of Early Recovery is the emergence of what people in AA call "character defects." During their drinking, many people become dishonest with themselves and others and increasingly defended in the service of maintaining denial. Many of the defenses and defects become visible and even magnified in recovery because there is such an emphasis on honesty. Families often hope that everything will be wonderful and are horrified when negative behaviors and defenses continue in recovery. Cal Girard illustrates:

"I was still a liar in recovery, just a sober, controlling liar. I couldn't tell Jean the whole truth so I'd give her half and I felt good about that. I thought she should be proud of me because I was trying and a half-truth was better than a whole lie. But she was more devastated to know I'd lied. I had always lied about everything. Telling the truth has been the hardest part of recovery."

Once again, we've emphasized the hard road and the difficulties people have. But that's not to say that Early Recovery isn't quite wonderful for many people, especially when the intense craving lessens or is gone completely. Lots of our interviewees have told us it was a time of great excitement, wonder, and awe. With 29 months of abstinence, Glen Russell says he's gotten a new life:

"I've come awake; out of the haze. I can listen to others and respond, so we're talking a lot now. Plus I've got all kinds of new interests."

But nobody says it was easy or that it came naturally. Everybody says it takes work and it takes a commitment. Bill Graham, whom we encountered in Chapter 9, summarizes the changes he's made:

"Early on, I'd storm out of the house and announce that I was going to a meeting. I'd be angry, explosive, and get everyone upset. My behavior was just as irresponsible and I thought I was just as special as I did when I was drinking. By about a year and a half, I'd gone from being special to accepting responsibility for acting normal. I went from a 'bad drunk' to a 'good drunk' and then from a 'recovering drunk' to a good, normal guy, parent, and husband. It was a 'dethroning.' I got a sense of myself in relation to other people by getting out of the center. I had to be able to see and hear my wife. I had to be responsive and available. I had always been undependable. These changes are still occurring [at 8 years]."

The Coalcoholic in the Early Recovery Stage

The task for the partner and family in Early Recovery is to build and solidify a new identity and behaviors that accompany abstinence. It is a time to strengthen the processes of disengagement and detachment from the alcoholic and the alcoholic family system and to learn to fill those needs in a different, healthier way, such as through active participation in Al-Anon. The partner continues to focus on the self in this process of individual exploration and growth. Karen Graham illustrates:

"I went to Al-Anon for 3 years before Bill stopped drinking, and it was 2 years before I gave up the idea that I could get him to stop. It was hard to look at myself and impossible to do it alone."

Focusing on the self is very difficult for the person who has been vested in worrying about and trying to control the alcoholic. Many coalcoholics acknowledge that they do not have an experience of themselves, or even an identity, separate from that of "spouse"—the one responsible for everyone else. It is often harder for the partner to focus on the self than it is for the alcoholic who has typically been the center of attention during the drinking and early abstinence.

Daryl Innis, who always thought that alcoholism was his wife's problem, watched her change in recovery and began to think:

> "For awhile, I was glad just to see Elaine not drinking and I even thought that alcoholism was over for us! Then one day it struck me that there was an opportunity in this recovery process for me too. I had a wonderful awareness that I could make something of this turning point. I needed something for me."

Coalcoholics may continue to experience considerable fear and anxiety: fear that the alcoholic may drink again and fear of a different way of life (the AA or Al-Anon programs); guilt for prior behavior and guilt for all the feelings they have carried toward the alcoholic in the past and present. Many coalcoholics feel intense anger and resentment about all the trauma of active alcoholism and about the uncertainty of recovery. Many note that they "walked on eggshells" for years into recovery, still feeling controlled by the alcoholic—drinking or not. Many also worry about their children: what's happened to them in the past and what kind of repair is possible? Even those who develop strong Al-Anon programs worry. Pam Richardson, whom we met in Chapter 9, remembers:

> "I was addicted to Matt and couldn't stop worrying. I had to learn the difference between caring and addiction. I worried for three years into recovery and then I stopped. That was the end of my focus on him. I think he missed it at first. I stopped reacting, and I think it upset him. I had found myself and my own recovery. I couldn't worry about him anymore."

Early Recovery is a time of great individual change. Coalcoholics work the 12-step program and, as Karen Graham says, face their own character defects: "I was angry and had carried it all for years."

Coalcoholics may feel ineffective in the marriage. They may feel a general uneasiness in the company of other couples, as well as envy and jealousy of others who do not have to deal with alcoholism. They may feel scared of relapse, scared of recovery, and helpless to control the relationship. Sometimes they wish things would go back to "normal" (they mean back to drinking). Sherry Robinson remembers:

"I was more independent and had more self-esteem when Alan was drinking. I was in charge of things, and I took care of him. When he got sober, he was gone a lot and I missed him. I felt the loss for a long time."

Regardless of whether coalcoholics are in recovery, they may feel neglected, abandoned, and competitive with AA. Coalcoholics may experience anger at themselves for staying with the alcoholic, anger at the alcoholic for past drinking behavior, or anger at the outside world generally. Coalcoholics may feel distrustful, unforgiving, and fearful.

Jean Girard recalled the early years:

"I went to Al-Anon for Cal and resisted it for a long time. I was addicted to him and I had to recognize it, but I couldn't till he left. I was in agony. He had been my lifeline. We separated at 1 year of recovery.

"He had affairs when he was drinking, which I refused to see. When I learned he had had affairs in recovery, I hit bottom. It was excruciating. How much further could this go? I was a sucker.

"In this period I was catatonic. I wasn't a good parent; I lost all judgment. I left our daughter in front of the TV for hours and days. I had no resilience left and thought of killing myself.

"I found a new Al-Anon home group and the best sponsor. I couldn't accept myself, but they could and did. It took awhile, but I became filled with a sense that I'm OK.

"After a year, we decided to live together again. Then Cal slowly told me the truth—I didn't get it all till several years into recovery. It's been a long hard road. I had to grow a lot and find myself. We have made it so far, and our relationship is strong and growing."

Though Early Recovery is hard, many coalcoholics—worried or not—are also deeply grateful, relieved and full of hope about recovery. Ron Baxter (whom we met Chapter 8 and 9) recalls what it was like:

"There are degrees of change. The first years are the hardest. You can't ever take anything for granted. Deb started taking responsibility for herself, which was a big change for a caregiver like me. I had to step back and learn to let go. As a manager, I was paid to help people feel better and work together. Going to Al-Anon helped me see what was and what was not my responsibility. The next few years were full of compromise, which was very hard. At some point, we had to make a decision to be separate and equal. We did it. But we never could have done it without recovery. We would have gone our separate ways. We are so grateful to have come so far."

Looking back, with 9 years of recovery, Denise Castle (whom we met in Chapter 9) recalls the powerful changes she made early on:

"We stayed out of each other's way. I became committed to my own recovery and stopped keeping track of his. At first, if Tony didn't go to AA, I wouldn't go to Al-Anon. But not anymore. My attitude change was as big as his not drinking."

The Children in the Early Recovery Stage

The experiences of children in Early Recovery are as varied as their particular family histories and circumstances of recovery. For some, Early Recovery is great: safe, secure, with parents available, and life feeling much, much better. For others, it's not so hot.

As we've said, interest in the family system ranks behind the parents' focus on their individual recoveries—that is, if all goes well. In some families, interest in the well-being of children may also rank below the parents' recoveries. We said earlier that what is best for the parents and for the long-term health and well-being of the children and family—the focus off of the system and onto the individuals—is not necessarily good for the children in the short term. Nor is it necessarily bad. It depends on many factors: the ages of the children; how much they have been told about the reality of alcoholism as it was happening in the past and as recovery has progressed; and how much they can be included or want to be included in Early Recovery. Every one of our research families was different in this respect. Some kids loved recovery, and some hated it. Some wanted to be involved, and others couldn't get far enough away. Most were glad about abstinence but didn't want it to interfere with their needs. As Jane and Len Irving (above) put it, "The kids looked at us as if we were crazy. We were talking this new language and all wrapped up in ourselves. Several times they told us, 'Fine, but what about us?'" Other kids tried hard not to be a burden to their suffering, needy parents who were so new to recovery.

There remains a serious danger that children will be neglected and abandoned if both parents are enthusiastically committed to and following their individual programs of recovery. They may be neglected and abandoned if one parent is in recovery and the other is not. And they may be abandoned if no one seeks help outside the family. Parents may be no better able to attend to their children in Early Recovery than they were during the Drinking or Transition stages, regardless of the status of their individual commitment and growth.

We said it earlier; we'll say it again. We hope that parents will never be forced to choose between their sobriety and their children. Yet we understand the conflict families face: we do not believe that a parent's recovery should ever supersede the needs of a child, yet we know it happens all the time as the parents' need to maintain abstinence must be the highest priority. In the real world, attending to both individual recovery and to the best interests of children can be very difficult. We know it is hard, and we want to acknowledge how difficult it is so that it can be addressed. Making sure that children are not lost to recovery is everybody's business. Holly Davis (above) talks about her sense of loss:

"There was a lot of chaos and confusion in the first 2 years as Mom was steeped in recovery. But I expected that I'd have her back after a while: there was no more drinking and I could relax. Then how come I felt so bad for 3, 4, and 5 years? I asked myself, 'How come I'm feeling as bad as I do? How come things aren't right and don't fit together? How come Mom never comes home?' I was so lonely. And angry. She'd done what I wanted—stopped drinking. Now I was in need of a Mom and she wasn't around."

The Davis family has continued to live in crisis for years into abstinence. Tension still dominates family life as everybody argues about who, besides Mom, is alcoholic. Mom is worried about Dad and several of the children. Dad and the kids maintain that Mom is the only problem. Mom is abstinent, but the family remains deeply angry and divided. Mom tells us there are two leaders, herself and her husband, but she adds that neither of them can really lead. Both defer to the children: "Someone makes pronouncements and everybody reacts. Nobody ever agrees, and decisions aren't acted on. It ends up that the person who wants it just does it."

Here we see a continuation of the drinking environment and system. There is chronic tension with much ongoing hostility. This is a family that has stabilized in a war-zone atmosphere. The system is structured to reinforce chaos—too many leaders and no one leads. It's a "save yourself" kind of world.

Theoretically, individual recovery is not bad for the kids; but, in the worst case, the traumatic experience of Early Recovery can be parents who are angry, scared, moody, arguing, threatening, out of control, or totally absent. So, it's important for adults to consider the needs of their children as they reorganize their lives around all of the action and new learning of the individual recovery focus. Educational support groups for children of alcoholics can be very helpful as a way of extending the individual focus to include the children, without shifting to a family systems view. As we said in Chapter 9, the younger the children the more likely that they can be included in the development of a newly recovering family. Preadolescents and teens may need to resist the pull back into a newly abstinent family since their normal process of separation from the family is usually underway. They may feel regret and anger at the loss of their parents to recovery because they need their parents' full attention and support for launching into adulthood. Some of the teenagers in our research have become the new identified alcoholics in the family; others express worry about their drinking. For example, 17-year-old Ginger Jacobson tells us and her parents that she wants to drink all the time and is scared to death. "I don't want to become an alcoholic," she says.

Ala-Kid and Alateen can be especially helpful for children and adolescents, respectively. These groups normalize feelings and provide peer support in dealing with the reality of alcoholism and the problems of both drinking and recovering parents. Children and adolescents will learn that they didn't cause the problems and the danger of isolation will be reduced. Children will also learn how to cope with family reality.

The teenagers in our study had mixed feelings about Alateen. Many found it to be helpful and supportive, and they loved having a part in family recovery. Others were scared by the stories they heard. They believed their own families were not nearly as bad as what they were hearing in Alateen meetings, and so they resisted identifying with the other teens. Some told us they hated all the meetings and all of recovery. There was so much change to deal with and so much to be anxious about, particularly the threat of a parent's relapse. Many of these youngsters grew to like recovery a lot as time passed and a parent did not drink. Kids, like adults, don't want to feel needy, vulnerable, or open to someone who can suddenly become drunk and leave them shattered.

Sometimes children believe that they should not express anger, hurt, or any other painful feelings because the alcoholic is suffering from a disease. It is difficult to justify anger at someone who is sick. Yet anger is what they feel, along with a myriad of other emotions. Kids often feel terribly guilty: they believe that they caused the drinking before and they've caused the trauma afterward by simply being children who have needs (Black, 1981; Moe, 1995).

Just as in the Transition stage, during Early Recovery (or at any time) children need to feel safe and protected. When parents move out of the crisis of Transition and can tell their children what is happening in age-appropriate terms, the children also need to be seen and heard—and, we hope, nurtured.

Children of any age may experience the transformation or loss of family structure—new rules, roles, boundaries—as difficult, especially since parents are not focused on the family now in the same way that the kids still are and need to be. Although the parents are more or less cushioned against such jolts through AA and Al-Anon, they need to attend to putting new basic structures in place in order for their kids to feel the sense of safety and security they need.

The Russell family (above) no longer has teenagers—their three children are all grown—but they are in many ways living as a family with teens. Several of our families with grown children reported the same experience. Children who had missed the safety and closeness of parents and home when they were adolescents often come back home "to do it again" when their parents are in recovery. These grown children in their 20s and 30s tell us that it is wonderful to be going back home. The environment feels safe, and they love the newfound access to parents. This is a good example of the solid change in the environment and family system that many families find by Early Recovery, or at least in the period of 3–5 years of abstinence.

Jane and Len Irving (above) say that their kids, who were just leaving home when Jane stopped drinking, now come home regularly for an ice cream social. These parents and kids were never together like this during their childhood years. Kids who missed parental attention and engagement growing up are hungry for it now, no matter how old they are.

Holly Davis (above) still wants her mother to pay attention. But she sees that the roles are now just as reversed as they were during the drinking: "My mom is always screaming for attention, and I don't want to give it to her."

Grown children also like what they see. In several of our research families, adult children are also in recovery, for their own addictions, and/or they are involved in Al-Anon. Charlie King says he reacted positively to his mother's recovery after the initial shock of abstinence:

"I loved what I saw happening for her, and I wanted to learn from her example. I went to Al-Anon too and learned to set limits for myself. It's been the best thing that's happened to me. I also go to AA. I love to listen to the stories and am so moved by people's honesty."

The Robinson children, Andrea, 19, and Owen, 15, highlight the positive evolving experience of Early Recovery:

ANDREA: I didn't like my father after recovery. I couldn't trust him, and he was an ass. Before I could get away with anything, and now he was telling me what to do. I liked having only one parent, so I just blocked him out. He tried to jump back in and be my dad, and I didn't want it. It took me a year to let him in, and then I started to like him. But I stayed angry too; I kept a wall up as I watched. I was afraid I'd be hurt.

One time in the first few months I was embarrassed because a friend saw the AA meeting book on the counter. She told me her mother was in AA too! I couldn't believe it. I began to write all of my papers about alcoholism, and I even wrote a poem for my father. It was hard. I didn't want him to know I cared so much. My most important feeling now is that I can rely on him. After 3 years, it's wonderful.

OWEN: My father wanted to include me right away. He was a real Dad, we got close and it was scary. I thought he might be drinking. Before, when he stopped, I felt real close and then he drank. I heard yelling, and Andrea was crying. I realized he must be drinking again. I hated it. So this time I didn't want to get burned. I talked to my mom all the time—still got information from her and stayed scared. I watched and listened to him at dinner. I'm not sure when I started to feel more confident and less afraid—maybe after a year. He went to meetings every day, and it felt good. Nothing went wrong at my junior high graduation. The last two years have been better and better. I have a lot more trust. We have a good, close relationship, and it's easier to talk. I can ask him things now instead of being scared.

So, Early Recovery is a mix: it's wonderful, because there is some stability and some trust in recovery; but it's still so new that parents may be unavailable and more self-focused than the kids would like or need. As we go next to Ongoing Recovery we will finally see the rewards of all the long, hard work of change.

CHAPTER ELEVEN

Ongoing Recovery for Couples and Families

W ell, is it ever going to slow down, calm down? Will things ever become stable, predictable, consistent? Will the hard work pay off? Is there a "there" to get to?

Our research families with many years of recovery have told us that, yes, things slow down and calm down and, yes, they become stable, predictable, and consistent. Definitely, yes, the hard work pays off, but is there a "there" to get to? No, in the sense that families don't ever arrive at an end point and they are never finished. Ongoing Recovery is a process, not an outcome. But everything does change, and so much is better.

There is no stable recovery without the passage of time. But time alone does not guarantee that individuals and family will be in the process of Ongoing Recovery. It's like the distinction AA members make between being "dry" and "sober." "Dry" refers to the state of abstinence—it's the "outcome"—while "being sober" refers to growth, change, and the quality of life (Brown, 1985). Families who are in Ongoing Recovery have experienced the developmental process of recovery. They can look back and tell a story of hard work and change. Other families stopped drinking, but there is no story to tell and no present that is any different from the past. Their recovery refers to a length of abstinence but not to a process of change.

It's important to remember that "looking good" is not necessary to healthy recovery. Sometimes "looking good" indicates an absence of growth and change. We expect that families in healthy recovery will have problems. What they've gained is the ability to deal with all that comes their way—past and present—in mature, respectful, and responsible ways.

OVERVIEW

The environment becomes very sure, safe, and protected. It now holds a security and often a comfort that used to be chaos and terror. Families told us they don't live in a magic wonderland but they do trust that the best and the worst of things will work out, and this is what happens. Although there may be crises, which are part of normal life, the family does not lose its basic core of security in dealing with whatever life brings. For example, Karen Graham (whom we met in Chapters 9 and 10) tells us her family had coped with the death of her father, a severe illness for Bill, her husband, and an economic hardship, all between 5 and 8 years of recovery. People had felt loss, grief, fear, anger, which they acknowledged and discussed. It was safe enough to feel and to deal openly with each crisis. The family environment never felt out of control.

The therapist knows that the environment of Ongoing Recovery can maintain its safety. Whether it does or not is a critical question in assessing the family with long-term abstinence. In Early Recovery too much trauma may lead to a chaotic, out-of-control experience that is partly a still-automatic return to a drinking state of mind and family atmosphere.

But by Ongoing Recovery, the environment does not become chaotic and out of control, despite unknowns and a lot of emotion about many things—the goods and the bads. The recovering family environment now "holds" the individuals, who live, love, work, play, and cope together.

Finally, the family system has settled into its new structure: partners are much more equal than not equal; rules and roles are clear and appropriate—parents are the parents and kids are the kids; boundaries are clear but also flexible; and communication is open and honest, and things make sense. The adults, who have long been so focused on their individual development, can now come back together to focus on the "we" of the couple while not losing the hard-won "I." "Separate and together" becomes a reality. Two individuals can now build a new healthy couple relationship based on the separateness, the individuality, and individual responsibility each has claimed and developed over the years of recovery. The strength of a healthy, cohesive system as well as solid individual growth keep the environment calm in the face of problems. A therapist working with a family with long-term recovery assesses the environment and system on all these dimensions.

And the individuals? Many report a deep gratitude for the gifts of sobriety. Most tell us they wouldn't change a thing, though the road was not easy. But they woke up, and they get to be awake for life. That means awake to all the pain and the pleasure; it means the right to be honest and the duty and responsibility to work things through. It means "showing up." So many adults and grown children express the view that, with help and sobriety, they have gotten a second chance to grow up and find themselves.

By Ongoing Recovery people trust the process, themselves, and each other. They know "it works" (an AA and Al-Anon slogan) if they maintain their individual programs and attachment to recovery. By now the therapist can hear gratitude and the solidity of healthy selves that shape the environment and system.

Is it all rosy? No. Does every family make it if people just stop drinking? Unfortunately, no. Some families live in pain, unhappiness, and even despair. We've given you plenty of examples so far. One major source of pain for families in Ongoing Recovery is a mismatch in commitment to individual growth—the couple in which one person is moving in recovery and the other is not. This difference in commitment to individual change was the single most important factor in determining the couples' and families' experience of closeness and well-being after 5 years of abstinence.

In the mismatch, partners struggle. One wants something from the other that the other can't or won't give. In several of our couples, partner A, the identified alcoholic, wanted partner B to say that he or she was also alcoholic but partner B wouldn't do it. The difference sometimes organizes everything in recovery so the couple can't go around it. There is tension and mistrust as couples struggle to establish closeness on a foundation of different realities. Growth can only go so far.

In such cases, a therapist would reflect these struggles back to a couple and wonder what purpose is served by couples continuing to differ so strongly. What would it be like if they solved these problems and if they found a base for greater trust? Sometimes these questions elicit a tremendous fear of intimacy, feelings and memories from the past, or other problems in the present that are harder to face than maintaining the distance and arguing about differences.

Other couples establish a ground for intimacy on a shared agreement to go around certain issues that threaten them. Some couples mention a fear of anger or sexual difficulties as unresolved issues that the couple had set aside, sometimes permanently. If the tabling involves stored up emotions, unnamed and unresolved, it may become a barrier to a full and free exchange. In some cases, it may not. Couples learn to circumvent all kinds of things as they adjust to each other's needs and wishes. Not dealing with things can be OK and even right. Not dealing with things that then must be hidden, and walked over and around, limits the depth and freedom of intimacy that is possible for partners.

Some couples get stuck in an unequal relationship or in unhealthy roles and rules that they cannot budge. The status quo works, though it may not work well. But it's too threatening to challenge, particularly since the alcoholic is abstinent. Opening up to change may very well scare both partners: what if it leads to drinking or the end of the relationship?

The therapist may say all of this to a couple seeking help. What happens if they start to budge the system? Are individual recoveries strong enough to tolerate more intensive couples work?

Something else causes pain for people in recovery: issues, feelings, and the realities of the past. Here, we're referring not only to what happened during the drinking but also back to childhood. What was it like growing up? Many people told us that they undertook a second "recovery" process—individually—somewhere past 5 years of abstinence. About 7 or 8 years of recovery seemed to be a target time, that is, if the issues and the pain of the past had not come up earlier. For many, the trauma of Transition and Early Recovery involved facing the resurgence of the past that wasn't staying quiet early on, giving the individual a "honeymoon break," or "pink cloud."

This is what we call the "trauma" work, the deep, uncovering of the past—the naming of reality, what happened, and the remembering and reexperiencing of feelings. For some, it is a new depth of awareness and affect related to their drinking or codrinking histories. People may now feel a more complete experience of loss, sorrow, and grief. This depth of "trauma" work may also be related to a deepening in uncovering work, through the steps and/or psychotherapy. Individuals may struggle with deep, unconscious, or split-off internalized images and conflicts that have intruded into the conscious experience of self in recovery. Many individuals in our research, alcoholics and nonalcoholics, grew up with alcoholic parents in the same kind of out-of-control, chaotic environments that they then created, the same polarized, dictator systems, and the same distorted and disturbed individual realities. Now, with a firm base of abstinence and with tools to keep them "grounded" (i.e., staying abstinent), individuals tackle the past. Remember Kay Warner in Chapter 4. She faced the incest she had grown up with, and she could hear about and acknowledge incest in her own family. This was not exactly a choice. She didn't feel whole or complete in sobriety; in fact, she felt "not too much." She did not have the joy of living she knew was possible. Something was there that she needed to see and know.

Trauma work involves not only remembering and reexperiencing feelings. It also involves working through the beliefs, motivations, and affects—intrapsychic and interpersonal—that the individual held, and determining to what degree the person contributed to developing and maintaining pathology and to what degree the individual was enculturated into pathology and adapted to it in order to establish and maintain attachments. Both are important factors in understanding individual development and adaptation. In fact, they are rarely separate. Yet it is often very confusing and conflictual for the alcoholic and coalcoholic who are also ACOAs. What am I responsible for? What did I have a choice about? This sorting through process is the standard work of Ongoing Recovery.

For many ACOAs in our research, the alcoholism went back to grandparents and beyond. Being alcoholic or married to an alcoholic was not an aberration, not the deviant, gone-wrong kid. It was a passing of the torch, a legacy lived through. And it was a legacy that our families interrupted—stopped. These individuals did not have a healthy, nonalcoholic past to return to. Recovery was a "starting-from-scratch" proposition.

In Ongoing Recovery the therapist charts movement through the stages and domains, alert to all difficulties whether they are related to alcoholism or otherwise. As we've noted, many individuals and couples can now benefit from intensive psychotherapy to help with the past and the present. The foundation of abstinence, the tools of recovery, and the development of a strong sense of self enable people to tolerate a wide and deep range of emotion in the service of continued growth. The therapist watches for a continuing all-encompassing focus on alcohol, which at this point may be defensive, limiting further growth. Gloria and Cliff Larkin provide an example:

Whenever Gloria and Cliff, with 10 years' abstinence, felt a twinge of anger, they quickly shifted from a focus on the couple to the frameworks of their individual programs. This defused the anger and reassured them that they were safe and that neither would lose control. But now they recognize that they need to know the feelings, to express them, and to sort through perceptions, beliefs, behaviors, motivations, and defenses at work in their couple relationship. Dealing with anger does not mean making it go away.

Before we look at the domains of Ongoing Recovery, let's hear again from Denise and Tony Castle (whom we met in Chapter 9), now with 9 years of abstinence. As they begin to report on their overall experience as an "alcoholic couple" in recovery, both say that they have had big arguments over the years. Then they try to recall what they were about, but they can't remember. Throughout the interview, they check in with each other, disagreeing sometimes, perhaps correcting their views, while chuckling and touching each other affectionately. Denise says:

"Basically, we've agreed. The concepts of the 'program' have strengthened our relationship. We started discussing what we were learning in our aftercare programs, and we've been talking ever since. We did not have good communication before, but now we do. During the drinking, Tony was verbally abusive. His foul language was rampant, and he wasn't willing to listen to my opinions. Before, it was like living with a person who was slowly going insane, but I didn't realize it. You keep trying to work it out, and it doesn't work.

"We talk everything over now and we kind of fight. I want explanations, which he can't always provide. I'll get silent, and I may even carry a resentment for a while and feel sorry for myself, but I don't obsess about it. We are able to accept our different perceptions and feelings.

"Our intimacy has grown over the years, and the same with sex. They used to be linked, but that's less so now. When sex has been difficult, we can talk about it.

"I have experienced a major attitude change. I can see now that

Tony does things out of guilt—not so much against me—so things make sense. The biggy for me over all these years is dealing with my belief that sobriety would fix everything.

"We enjoy a lot of things together now that are not geared around drinking or not drinking. We have compromised a lot, on small things and big ones. I need people while Tony likes being alone, so we moved to a place where I could have access to Al-Anon, my women's group, and a community, and Tony could have a sense of a quieter, less urban life. It's worked well, but I was afraid at first. I took a job right away, even though I was officially retired, because people would have to talk to me. I got myself out there, so I didn't feel isolated. I knew I was going to be OK when somebody in the store recognized me. Tony was doing his own thing, I was doing mine, and we were doing ours together."

Even in Ongoing Recovery, Denise maintains her recovery environment and 12-step structure. She knows that continuing participation keeps her paying attention to herself so she does not become isolated or slip back into old patterns. She does not define health as the ability to do without support. On the contrary, plenty of consistent, structural support allows her to stay healthy. Tony adds:

"I agree that the concepts of the program have been really important to us. I have questions now that never would have occurred to me before because my perceptions have changed. I never understood enough to ask intelligent questions. It happens pretty often now that I ask Denise, 'when I say this, why do you feel that?' We talk back and forth."

Tony describes their ability to sustain a dialogue that includes feedback, a hallmark of mature relationship and communication skills. He also demonstrates the evolutionary individual growth accomplished by time and work in recovery.

"Occasionally I still have rage, a sudden fury, and then it's gone. It used to happen a lot, but now I use the 10th step [Continued to take personal inventory and when we were wrong promptly admitted it; Alcoholics Anonymous, 1952, 1955), so I don't let little things build. Sometimes I have depression and short panic attacks like I used to have constantly. When I was drinking I had severe agoraphobia—in fact, I took bourbon to a support group for agoraphobics! I still have some panic and still have sleep problems, but I'm able to deal with them all.

"Yes, we fight. In our last argument, we were both right. It was about driving. We often fight about that. We also fight about family—never agree on that. I used to believe that everyone had the same perceptions or they were wrong or crazy. I learned that people come to things in different ways. Now Denise and I will use our programs and often come up with the same conclusions."

Tony illustrates the development of new internal structure that permits less egocentrism, more differentiation and thus less need for defense. Next he describes a shift from a dichotomous relationship framework to a more equal, complementary process:

"When I was drinking I used to try to influence decisions. I always had a sense of urgency, so I demanded and manipulated to get my way. Now we try to reach agreement on big decisions. We're 'fine-tuning' that process."

The therapist hears the development of internal structure that leads to greater internal security and a reduction in impulse. Recall the progression of ego development: In Transition and Early Recovery, individuals substitute an immediate behavior for an impulse to drink. Then they begin to add language so that eventually they can talk about their feelings and impulses without needing to act them out. Tony illustrates:

"My slogan used to be 'Make things happen.' Now it's 'Let things happen.' I'm not as conscious of goals; I notice road signs and landmarks along the way. Day-to-day, all is well and I can handle the bad. I think of several stages for me. First I had to get to the point that I didn't want to drink. Then I developed the 'Let it happen' thing, and finally I am learning how to live life. Where did we miss out on how to live life? I was never educated in a philosophy of life. I've gotten that in AA."

The therapist hears the development of basic trust (Erikson, 1963; Bowlby, 1980) in Tony's ability to shift from a driving need to control himself and others to an ability to be part of a process that requires a tolerance of uncertainty. He illustrates the "holding" (Winnicott, 1953, 1960) function of AA that enabled him to engage in the repair and development of a healthier, more secure self.

Let's go now to the domains.

THE ENVIRONMENT

Finally, the context of daily life—the atmosphere, the mood, the felt sense of safety—is secure, predictable, and consistent. The usual atmosphere is friendly and open rather than anxious or hostile. The environment values, supports, and reflects abstinence and recovery.

Of the three domains, the environment showed the strongest changes in response to abstinence alone *and* to the changes occurring in the system and individual domains. The environment reflects the health of the system and the individuals in it. Trust comes from safety, which comes with consistency and predictability. None of these is possible in a family in which the system is in collapse and the individuals are out of control. Only when new rules, roles, and boundaries are clear and individuals are focused on themselves instead of what's wrong with everybody else can the environment be safe.

As we've seen, the environment begins to be a safer place in Early Recovery when the family is organized around recovery and there is some stability and predictability. It also grows in safety as a result of parents reaching outside the family for support. Of course, we've emphasized that this reaching out can just as easily maintain an unsafe environment if parents fail to pay attention to their children and their welfare in this time of tremendous chaos and change.

By Ongoing Recovery the environment has become a safe haven that exudes a welcome and a warmth. People begin to trust that things will not get out of control in the home. It's as simple as that. But what a dramatic change. In the family of Ongoing Recovery, people don't have to live in terror. While problems and crises arise, family members trust that parents can be counted on to provide continuous safety and to be responsible for dealing with whatever arises. Much of Early and Ongoing Recovery involves learning how to do this in their programs and in therapy. Pam and Matt Richardson (whom we last encountered in Chapter 10) describe it:

PAM: Our son is more comfortable bringing his friends home now, which he never did before because he was terrified. We're just a lot more predictable; everybody feels better about themselves. Our story is one of change and hope, though it's filled with painful circumstances. Everybody's gotten better.

MATT: The story of our family's recovery is one of assimilation and enculturation into recovery as a way of life. I see it as an evolutionary process. My father died from alcoholism at 52. My grandfather died an alcoholic. I'm 47, recovering, and have been in recovery for 8 years. Our eldest son is recovering, and he's 24. Our kids have a reference point that I didn't have. They've gotten better unconsciously—we don't have discussions over dinner; we don't sit down and talk about our story. We're doing it. We've got four generations of alcoholics, and each is recovering sooner. Our family story has to do with personal responsibility.

The family therapist helped Pam and Matt establish limits they could not even think about on their own, and the therapist offered continuing support in holding to them. This "imposed" structure paved the foundation for their own internal individual development and a healthier system structure later on. It also established a recovery culture before they were able to develop their own. They relied heavily on outside supports since they felt incapable of knowing how to help themselves or their children early on. Readers may remember that Pam and Matt both had individual recovery programs, individual therapists, and family therapy as they maintained abstinence and faced the addictions of their children.

Karen and Bill Graham (above), with 8 years of recovery, have coped with major illness—Karen developed cancer in Early Recovery—and behavior and adjustment problems with their children during these years. The environment has been permeated by the threat of loss and acting-up kids. Still, Karen and Bill said they felt secure and able to tackle and cope with all of these difficulties. It wasn't easy, and they often weren't a "happy family," but there was never a feeling that they wouldn't get through it. Karen describes a symbol of the evolving trust:

"We recently sold our family home; it was a long, hard decision, because we'd lived there all our married life. There were holes in the walls—punched through in an angry rage—that reminded us what it used to be like. That home held all the realities and memories of drinking. We got ready to let them go. We've got a home now with few walls at all. And we laughed as we agreed to purchase new furniture—sofas with connecting pieces that can be separated or joined together in one big hunk. We all see this furniture as a symbol of the changes we've made. Our environment now allows us to be close, to flop together on the sofas, or to get a little more room. Before, we were literally walled off from each other."

Bill adds:

"Today we act normal. We listen and resolve things. We work and eat regularly. It's predictable and comfortable."

THE SYSTEM

The Family in the Ongoing Recovery Stage

The foundation for a healthy family system is in place. Parents have, or are working toward, a capacity to focus on the family and not lose their newly won healthy individual selves in the process. Testing this capacity to hold both perspectives is a major focus of daily life. New rules, roles, and boundaries are in place, or their development is firmly underway. These provide healthy structure in which deeper and more complex individual and couple growth can occur. Parents have shifted from an extremely polarized relationship during the drinking to a more equal partnership. Couple and parental decision making now reflects cooperation—shared input and responsibility. Open, direct, and honest communication can now take place.

This is the "best of all worlds" system. Some families get the best. In our research, it was usually the families in which both partners actively pursued their separate, individual recoveries and came back together with individual autonomy as the foundation of their new system and new relationship. This is what Denise and Tony Castle (above) did: two recoveries, separate at first and then separate and together.

Many families do it differently and also achieve a healthy, satisfying system that works. Other families do it differently and the system doesn't change at all, or it becomes arrested in an acceptable status quo but one that cannot grow (Steinglass et al., 1987). In the latter case, the structure isn't flexible enough, or the partners have become stalled in their individual growth, which keeps them and the system from changing. Often, trauma from the past is in the way and needs to be addressed by individuals or the family as a whole. The Smathers family provide an example. Mom and Dad both grew up in alcoholic homes, which they recognize but have not addressed. They then re-created the same kind of alcoholic family each had known. Now, Dad pleads with Mom and the kids to follow him in recovery. They say no. Neither the trauma of their childhoods nor the trauma of their own alcoholic past can be dealt with by anyone.

In recovery for 9 years, the Smathers family has fought the entire time. Dad wants everyone to be organized around recovery, and everyone else wants none of it. He is concerned about the kids' drinking, and he wants Mom to "get her own program." Dad wanted to participate in our research so he could try—yet again, in the opinion of family—to convince the others to join him in this new life. What an impasse! The other family members told us that there was chronic trauma during the drinking and it had continued unabated. Father was a dictator then, and he was still trying. During the interview, Dad is quite dominant, trying to exercise control over everyone. When his son points this out, Dad becomes sad and says:

> "All of recovery has been hard. I am powerless over the debris in this family. We still live in crisis after crisis, and we are incapable of dealing with anything."

It is important to remember our caveat: there are as many varieties of new family systems as there are families. The differences often work very well for people, so it is important not to draw conclusions about health, stability, or well-being of the system based on its pattern alone. Some couples who are successful in the emotional separation never find a path back together. Of those who do find that path, most have worked hard to get there.

The new family system is most often organized around recovery. Sometimes one individual leads the way in reorganizing the system. Other family members accept the changes and that person's leadership and don't get in the way. They are all receiving the benefits of recovery and adjusting positively in response to the changes in others. But they are not themselves in recovery. That may or may not come. Perry Mitchell describes it:

"We all admire our stepfather so much. He came into this family and saw what none of us could see. Over time, he led the way into recovery for all of us. Mom stopped drinking, and all of us have changed."

Jeremy Norton provides another example:

"Before recovery, there was nothing but chaos. We didn't have anything in common, or anything that felt like 'family.' Now recovery is a family organizing principle. We all relate around it. Nobody's in a program but Mom, but we all follow her lead."

Karen and Bill Graham (above) have a difference of opinion about how important the recovery focus should be. Bill says he doesn't want to be a "recovery junkie" and likes the broader life he has. He doesn't want to relate everything back to his alcoholism. He also told us that he has reaped the benefits of Karen's growing autonomy. Bill thinks that seeing themselves as a "recovering family" still puts too much emphasis (and blame) on him. They both participated in the drinking system and they've both contributed to recovery.

Karen doesn't disagree, but she wants a lot more involvement in recovery than Bill does at this point, 8 years in. So she continues to pursue her own program more actively than Bill does now, and together they have faced a lot of "old baggage" in couples therapy.

Sober for 11 years, Ginny Oldman lives with Marv, her husband, in a polarized system, focused on their continuing disagreement as to whether Marv is also an alcoholic. She has organized her life around her recovery and wants desperately to share a couple's life also organized around recovery. Marv, however, has organized his life around resisting her: he maintains that he is not an alcoholic and will not change his view. Ginny says she longs for the day when Marv will say he is an alcoholic; he only has to say it once; that's all she wants. Marv says no, never.

Ginny and Marv disagree about most things. They have achieved a *selective* process of agreement and support in their shared commitment to be good parents. Whenever the interests of their children are the issue, they work extremely well together, able to solve problems, compromise, and not get caught in emotional struggles. They agree that they share little intimacy, though they love each other and have no thought of separating. Ginny thinks back to her first few months of abstinence:

> "I have no name for what happened. I felt confused, in a fog, and I was unable to function. I knew there was a big change in the wind, and I wanted him to come with me. I needed him to acknowledge being alcoholic. I said to myself: 'I will drag you with me or lose you.' Since then, I've been in recovery alone. At first it was hard and I didn't think I could do it. But now we're on the same path. There's a space between us, but we're going in the same direction."

Ginny tells us that becoming abstinent was a declaration of her autonomy, which frightened her. Being in recovery lets her maintain her autonomy, while she also struggles to hold on to her husband. This couple went from a system in which they both drank to one in which Ginny was the identified alcoholic. Neither now consider Marv's current drinking a problem, though Ginny still wants him to say he is an alcoholic. Both have changed over time. They have a positive undercurrent in their couple bond, though they continue to disagree about most things. We think that Ginny and Marv may have conflicts regarding dependency, separation, and autonomy.

The development of healthy parents and a healthy system offers children the opportunity for much needed direct parenting including attention, guidance, support, and modeling. Young children may experience a safety unknown at any previous time in their lives and resume childhood development in this healthier context. Older children may return home, also seeking the emotional repairs and rewards of this healthier environment and system. Many of our families reported that they had provided therapy for their children at various points during recovery, and many had also sought couples and family therapy.

The Putnams, Dina, Trent, and their daughter Kendra, at 12 years of recovery, describe the changes in the family, beginning with Early Recovery when they had no system in place and nothing positive from the past to call on.

DINA: I had no input about anything early in our marriage. The wife does what the husband wants. If he disagreed with anything I said,

I gave in. So I couldn't do anything early on. I stayed out of his way.

TRENT: I was into conflict avoidance. I didn't want her to drink—that's all. I had no feelings a lot of the time, and I was overwhelmed with feelings. I was totally traumatized. Neither of us would make a decision about anything. We were both afraid. We lived with the "let things happen" model. Somehow, dinner gets on the table, shopping gets done. But you live in a fog and don't discuss any of it. You can go for years without making a decision.

Listening, Kendra offers, "I'm beginning to wonder if my tuned-out self was because of all this. There was nothing holding it together."

DINA: Now we're a normal family. We have cohesive time together and important similarities. We all like to read, and watch movies together. Every Sunday night is family. We spend a lot more time with the kids. We wanted a family that works, and we got it. It's really gotten better in the last 2 to 3 years. We've worked on communication and decision making. I no longer automatically give in, but I also don't have to fight just for the principle of it. That's how it felt to me early on. I just had to resist going along with Trent or I was giving in.

Dina and Trent spent almost 10 years with a partially collapsed system and a predominant emphasis on separation and differentiation. Only then were they able to begin to work together effectively on couple issues.

Dina and Trent had two children after Dina stopped drinking. They call them their "recovery kids." The family talks about having two completely different "family stories." Dina, Trent, and Kendra lived with the trauma of alcoholism and the distress of recovery. They still know it and share it. Alex and Haley, the younger kids, now 5 and 7 years old, know that Mom goes to meetings, but they don't know "recovery" and they don't talk "recovery." Their development will be shaped by a very different environment, system, and parenting than their older sister experienced. They will not grow up under the same influence of chaos and chronic trauma that Kendra knew. They may have other issues and problems to deal with, but the building blocks that enable healthy development are in place for them. They have the opportunity to learn healthy coping rather than unhealthy adaptation and defense.

Haley and Alex chat with us about school and their admiration for Kendra. Both agree that their favorite time is Sunday when the family is together. They giggle as they describe the months-long process the family engages in every fall. Each person gets to advocate his or her choice for the vacation destination the next summer. They gather information, each presents his or her "case," and the family votes. Everybody gets to win at some point. All agree that this is happy time. Haley proudly tells us that she won last year and the prize was Disneyland. The others agree they had a great time. This was a family in which the parents couldn't talk to each other for the first 2 years of abstinence.

Several of our research families emphasized the importance of rituals in the family's life (Steinglass et al., 1987; Wolin et al., 1979). In the past, rituals may have been a part of drinking, so that the family's sense of itself—its identity—was marked and reinforced by drinking. Stories of ACOAs make this painfully clear: memories of holiday times ruined by drunken parents; excited anticipation of birthdays and other special times replaced by the expectation of disappointment.

Early in recovery, everyone may fear holiday time because it awakens the memories and all the pain of drinking. It will take time to establish new rituals that are unhitched from drinking and all the horror that went with it. Some families begin by establishing rituals related to recovery, such as AA, Al-Anon, Alateen, or Ala-Kid birthdays—30 days, 60 days, 1 year, and on. In this way, the parents bring their new recovering identities into the family. This is of course easier to do if other members of the family are also in recovery, or at least supportive of it. In some families the last thing people want is new rituals linked to recovery. People may still be too angry, hurt, and resistant. This may be especially true for teens who, at first, are likely to have very mixed feelings about all the change and uproar of recovery.

In some drinking families, rituals have been protected from drinking instead of being absorbed by the alcoholic focus (Steinglass et al., 1987; Wolin et al., 1979; Wolin & Bennett, 1984) These families may be able to carry the rituals from the past into recovery without skipping a beat, thus providing consistency and continuity of positive family relationship to the otherwise very disrupted time of Transition. Wolin and his colleagues suggest that ritual preservation during drinking is a significant factor in resilience of children. Karen Graham (above) provides an example:

> "We placed a high value on traditions and rituals, so I was quite insistent on continuing them, or at least the ones that we could keep without upsetting anybody. We always had special family dinners, with candlelight and favorite foods, that we continued, with some modification. We loved these times, even though we had some problems over the years because of drinking. It wasn't too hard to maintain these occasions in recovery and build in the excitement of the old and the new. Once in a while one of us got too anxious or upset, because it reminded that person of all we'd been through. But that gave us a chance to deal with it—to remember the past and to really recognize how far we'd come. So it was mixed. We think these dinners, and the fact we all worked hard to continue this tradition, were a very helpful, stabilizing ritual for us in the drinking and in recovery. Now, they're a time for rejoicing at how far we've come and the closeness we feel."

The family's healthy development will be influenced by each person. For example, the presence of severe developmental difficulties related to being the child or ACOA (as so many of our adults were), intense internal conflict, or chronic personal or marital problems for the adults can mean a rougher road for family recovery. The growth of the system influences the individuals as much as they influence the system. Differences in rate of recovery by the parents or a continuing crisis-dominated environment and system complicate or retard individual growth within the family as well as the family system's recovery as a whole.

The success family members have had in obtaining help throughout the recovery process will also make a difference. Many families who have utilized external resources to work through the tasks of the early stages will experience Ongoing Recovery as an expansive period in which the family can begin to meet interpersonal needs more effectively.

Others may feel threatened by the possibility or expectation of greater intimacy or expansiveness in relationship. Often, unresolved trauma and internal conflicts surface now. Defenses against openness and closeness, helpful in warding off or easing anxiety in Early

Recovery, may now interfere. In Ongoing Recovery, the therapist can be helpful in questioning or challenging defenses focused on separation or differentiation rather than routinely supporting them.

The Couple in the Ongoing Recovery Stage

The mechanics and basic skills of family functioning are now in place. Couples have a new ability to problem solve. Now more equal than polarized, they are able to be flexible and adaptable. New rules, roles, and boundaries lay the foundation for the couple to actively explore and deepen their communication that will enhance their intimacy. It is time, often the first time, for the couple to become a "we" *and* two "I's." But this is not easy. In fact, some couples are so frightened of "intimacy" that they delay or avoid expanding their attention from their individual recoveries to include the couple. One of the reasons for delay is the fear by both of "loss of control." Many couples are terrified of opening up a dialogue in which they relinquish control of the content, the flow, and the outcome. Dialogue means "back and forth," a foray into "who knows what." In fact, couples often can tackle very tough subjects, but they don't realize it. The fear of loss of control dominates. As we noted earlier, several of our couples told us they remained afraid of talking about sex and anger, two topics that can become "out of control" in discussion or in the experience. "Loss of control" is still so dangerous because people fear that the emotional experience of openness may be too close to the memories linked to the loss of control of drinking. This is not an unrealistic fear! Even in Ongoing Recovery people may still experience a hangover following a sexual encounter, an angry exchange, or a fun time. Coalcoholics are reminded of drinking and their own reactions to it by a partner's increased emotional experience and expression, which may be quite positive, the result of deeper self-exploration. Drinking dreams, so common for people in recovery, often signal an opening up of emotion (which is expected in recovery), though they may also warn the individual of a real danger of drinking. Following an intense emotional experience in therapy, one individual said he could taste the scotch.

So, couples fear that the relinquishment of control will lead back to drinking. Some couples are afraid to raise delicate issues of any kind. They still fear naming certain feelings or issues because naming makes them real. What is real can become out of control. Or, at least, once a thing is named, people fear they cannot control the outcome. For example, a partner knew for a long time that the other was having an affair; but he said nothing, knowing that once he named the reality, he would have to take an action that might not lead to the outcome he wanted.

Couples worry that they will not be able to resolve the issue and, they reason, things will never be the same. But, again, their fears often outweigh the reality, though many don't test it out. Several of our couples described this process—walking a cautious couples path with many years of recovery—and the help they received with couples therapy. Both partners felt safer opening up difficult issues with the help of a third party. If the therapist knew something about recovery, so much the better. Certainly the therapist had to be supportive of recovery and understand the importance of the system's collapse and subsequent separation and differentiation. These couples needed help with each other; the focus was coming back into the home and onto their relationship.

Several couples with years of recovery could not establish a mature intimacy because they had not changed their system. The couple structure remained organized around old patterns of relationship. Roles, rules, and boundaries often didn't change. The individuals were abstinent, but their closeness was based on maintaining a parent–child bond. Les and Emma Quarles, with years of abstinence, illustrate.

Both believe that Les took care of Emma during the drinking and he took care of her when she stopped. She attended AA and developed a recovery program, but Les did not. Emma wanted him to participate in *her* recovery, which he willingly did. He "watched over" her, as an AA sponsor might, asking if she'd been to meetings, what step she was working, and how she was feeling. Both held the illusion that she would never be able to remain sober without him. Needless to say, it was threatening to both of them to consider separate programs and a focus on the self. Although Emma had maintained abstinence, she also felt anxiety when she contemplated making her own decisions.

The therapist addresses the function of this arrested system: Are these roles and rules still necessary? What would happen if Les stopped worrying about Emma and stopped monitoring her program? What would it be like for Emma?

Nate and Rita Randall have had a similar relationship. Sober for 10 years and secure in Nate's individual recovery in AA, they focused their couple relationship on his childhood trauma and depression. Both say they had a close partnership, but, as in the case of Les and Emma, it was based on the belief that Nste could not manage alone. They tell us their recovery was organized around coping with his depression, which dominated them both, just as alcohol had done for so many years.

This couple had reestablished a symbiotic system like the one they had during the drinking. As a result, they lost their footing in the individual recovery process. With couples therapy they could see that they had relinquished the autonomy each had gained in the first several years. The therapist helped them refocus on themselves and disengage from the organizing role of Nate's depression. They both recognized that they were frightened of giving up their overinvolvement with each other.

Neither of these couples could establish a healthy intimacy with its spontaneity and freedom of expression because one or both partners were suffering so much from the trauma of the past. They still needed too much control over themselves and others. Many of these people found individual therapy, ACOA or other kinds of group therapy, and/or couple therapy immensely helpful in addition to their recovery programs.

Brenda and Russ Sandburg report significant changes in their couple system over 7 years of recovery. Their changes were organized around abstinence and the couple therapy they had been in for almost 3 years. Although they did not belong to 12-step programs, they pursued individual recoveries through strong religious commitment and individual therapies. Both say they are not the same people who originally met each other.

Ron and Deb Baxter (whom we met earlier in Chapters 8, 9, and 10), with 17 years of sobriety, joke, with affection about needing each other's help more and more as they neared retirement. As Ron says, "Together, we are two 'half-brains.' " Then, seriously, they spell out the key ingredients of their couple focus now:

RON: It's always been hard to compromise, but that's what recovery has been about. We can disagree, and it's OK. Every year on Deb's sobriety anniversary we have a summit. We look at what we need to improve in our recovery—what do we want to focus on. This year, we'd like to be more forgiving. We've got the tools now of AA and Al-Anon, we've got the experience of others, and we've both found psychotherapy very helpful. We live in "Act III" now, between tiptoeing through the minefield and smelling the roses. We're at the time of life where we need to be supportive of each other. We spend time together, and we choose things we both enjoy. We have learned to play to each other's strengths.

DEB: A lot of our recoveries have been focused on individual things we don't share. That's why we pay attention to us together—so we don't develop parallel lives.

Deb and Ron say they have seen other recovering couples drift far apart to the point they had nothing in common. Ron and Deb decided early on to pay some attention to their couple bond—to not just forget about it or diminish the importance of their relationship in the interests of the individual focus.

Martina and Ryan Torres illustrate the long hard road. Ryan has been sober for 8 years, and both have been involved in individual recovery programs. They have lived in a "recovery model," as they put it, but up until last year their lives were just like drinking.

Martina says:

"We have lived through one trauma after another. First it was Ryan's PTSD [posttraumatic stress disorder] from Vietnam, then my own childhood living with two alcoholic parents. Then we faced problems with our kids. It's been a lot like drinking in the sense that it's been chaotic and very painful. It always seems I'm faced with powerlessness about something very hard."

What happened last year? Ryan says, "We began living a recovery norm, with less chaos and pain, when we got some couples therapy." They have also worked through significant individual trauma from the past so they are now free emotionally to strengthen their couple bond.

Karen and Bill Graham (above) talk a lot about spirituality and how vital it has been to both of them, both as individuals in recovery early on and now together as a couple:

BILL: It's the core of recovery and unique to each individual. Spirituality is necessary to a complete approach to recovery. When you take away the major method of coping—alcohol—you're left with a void. So you have to construct another way of coping. It's more than behavioral. It's emotional and spiritual. You have to believe in a Higher Power that allows you to get beyond yourself.

KAREN: I wanted spirituality so bad I could taste it. But I was angry at God for so long. And I couldn't be a representative of God with the dark side I carried, the anger and the jealousy. I had to get to the depths of that dark side, what keeps me from spirituality. I didn't want my unconscious creeping up.

A lot of people speak about the importance of spirituality in their recovery at all stages. Yet there may be great variation in what people mean by it. As we noted earlier, we think of spirituality as encompassing people's relationship to and acceptance of their fundamental human dependence. Addiction is dependence gone awry. The thinking disorder that maintains active addiction involves a denial of dependence. Many people in recovery and psychotherapy have come to terms with their need for help and thus the folly of their belief in self-sufficiency or self-power. In Ongoing Recovery, people are defining what healthy dependence means and working toward a balance between individual responsibility and interdependence. For many people in AA, healthy dependence involves a belief and trust in "a power greater than the self."

Finally, Len Irving (whom we've encountered above in Chapters 8, 9, and 10) sums it up:

> "During the drinking, we were like puzzle pieces that fit tightly together. Now, we are like loosely tied planets."

As a result of developing stronger individual selves, Jane and Len Irving have achieved a deeper level of trust and intimacy that has allowed them both separateness and togetherness in their relationship. Len continues:

> "There's been a progression in our relationship from mine and hers, to our house, to you and yours. It's evolved from I to me to us. Now, it's 'our' problem, which we can work on together."

INDIVIDUAL DEVELOPMENT

The Alcoholic in the Ongoing Recovery Stage

In Ongoing Recovery, everything is more stable in relation to alcohol and being alcoholic. The identity and the behaviors of abstinence have long been routine. Recovery actions and beliefs are solid and frequently the central organizing principle of the individual's life. Many people described living comfortable, very satisfying lives guided by recovery principles. Many also described concrete as well as internal changes.

Drew Underwood, sober 7 years, emphasizes the gains he has made:

> "I am thrilled with the changes. I used to have trouble remembering conversations, and I was having trouble keeping anything straight at work or at home. Now I can do more than one task and think about more than one thing at a time without forgetting things or becoming confused. And I have learned to listen. I used to listen to the first few sentences and then jump in with a solution."

Drew tells us that these changes within him have resulted in improved work relationships and a much better, more intimate relationship with his wife.

Alongside the comfort, deep gratitude, and even the joy of living comes an unexpected "opportunity." With abstinence solid, people can tackle other issues of all kinds. Some may awaken the past to face traumas from childhood and traumas related to their own drinking. This work is stimulated by working the 12-step program of AA, and it emerges through the normal course of living sober. People become "ready" to deepen their personal exploration. They may experience depression, anxiety, sleep difficulties or other addictions such as overeating, gambling or overspending that push them to question more deeply. As it did for Kay Warner (in Chapter 4), the past may push itself through, demanding acknowledgment. What has been forgotten, denied, or minimized can now be safely recognized and understood. Elaine Vernon illustrates:

> "In the beginning, I was working intensely on myself, though I thought it was terrible that I had to be so separate from my family. As I got emotionally sober, I did a lot of important work on my feelings about my children and about being an alcoholic mother. I could make amends for the emotional damage I had done and I had hope that they could get better. I had a shift in my thinking, almost like a spiritual awakening. One day I recognized the

uselessness of guilt and let go of it. Then my relationships began to change, and things have been different ever since."

This intensive uncovering process is never easy. But, if people stay sober a long time, they "become ready" to tackle more difficult work. Many individuals add psychotherapy to facilitate this process. It is paradoxical that longer sobriety can bring more pain. Of course, it also brings a great freedom, peace and stability never known before. Jill Fitzgerald, whom we met in Chapter 9 and who grew up with an abusive alcoholic mother illustrates:

"Alcohol has been the central theme of my life. I have learned in recovery that I don't have to do it all over again. I don't have to be an abusive wife and mother."

As we've seen, the trauma of the past may not wait till Ongoing Recovery to appear. Many people must struggle with all kinds of pain early on. Then and now, as other problems and symptoms emerge, a person may jump to the conclusion that "there must be something wrong with my program if I am having trouble." This is always difficult to sort through at any stage. It comes from a faulty belief, common to just about everyone, that abstinence and solid recovery should bring happiness, serenity, and inner peace. If people experience emotional pain, they and others often assume it's because they don't have a strong recovery or they are not "working the program" properly. Some people worry about "slacking off," and others become anxious at feeling so good. The emergence of other issues may automatically prompt relapse precautions. While it is a wise precaution at any time, in Ongoing Recovery a focus on relapse should be part of a larger picture, including the exploration of past and present issues and emotions that are now safer to experience. But the therapist should not jump to the conclusion that new anxiety means something is wrong or try to "fix" such difficult and uncomfortable feelings.

It is hard to accept that a good, solid recovery prepares people to face more difficult issues. It is exactly the opposite of "doing something wrong." But it rarely feels that way at first. New anxiety and feelings of being out of control that come with the unknown are usually threatening until the next level of work is revealed and people embark on a deepening process. Unfortunately, some people strengthen their defenses against new feelings or insights because of fear of what will emerge or of what others might say. Again, many people incorrectly assume that they are failing if difficulties emerge at this point in recovery. People may become more defended, more rigid and frightened. The great freedom and expansiveness in internal experience made possible by abstinence may itself cause new anxiety. With solid recovery and support, people can use this anxiety in the service of extraordinary personal growth. It is a turnaround from the past in which the automatic response to anxiety was alcohol.

Ironically, one of the major sources of anxiety is the couple relationship. Individuals are now ready to turn their attention back to the couple and to work on issues from the past while exploring their communication, openness, and capacity for intimacy in the present. We've stressed all the way through that relationships are difficult. Now is the time for a couple focus in addition to the individual focus. Yet this "opportunity" may initially cause people to strengthen their defenses, as the prospect of greater intimacy can be threatening. Recall what we said earlier: intimacy carries with it the threat of loss of control. All the work of Early Recovery now pays off: individuals have greater autonomy; relationships can be more equal; couples can engage in dialogue in which the course and outcome are unknown till they get there. But it's a lot to cope with.

How do people do it? Inherent to all the work we've described is the development of a personal understanding and relationship to spirituality, or what is known in AA as the "Higher Power." In Ongoing Recovery, an emphasis on spirituality is a central part of the deepening process for the individual and the couple. It may be part of the "trauma work," or it may be separate. People in AA have been in the process of exploring their "dependence" since the beginning, when they acknowledged the loss of control of their drinking and the need for help. Early on, they learned to substitute a recovery action for the impulse to drink, such as using the phone to contact an AA friend or going to a meeting, thus "depending on" the experience and example of others. Long-term sobriety brings a maturation in people's deepest sense of themselves and their reliance on "something greater." There is time for self-reflection. For some, this means continuing involvement with or returning to organized religion, as well as therapy, reading, going back to school, and other kinds of personal growth experiences. For others, it is a continuation of AA work and a deepening in the meaning of AA principles. For most, it's both.

People who do not belong to 12-step programs may experience a similar kind of deepening and personal growth, though not alone. Several individuals we interviewed have emphasized the importance of religion or psychotherapy. We feel most confident about AA since so many of the alcoholics in our research families belong to AA and testify to its importance.

The belief in and reliance on "something greater" helps the individual and the couple avoid returning to old, unhealthy beliefs and patterns of behavior. The belief in a "Higher Power" helps couples avoid struggles for dominance that can so easily crop up in close relationships where dependency is a key factor. When both partners invest their deepest dependence in something greater than the self *or the partner* (Brown, 1993), they are freed to establish an equal, interdependent relationship. It's not easy but possible. When a partner is elevated to the status of a "Higher Power," trouble invariably follows. Unhealthy dependence makes equality impossible.

Unchanged environments or unchanged family systems may continue to provoke great conflict to the degree that the alcoholic's identity and recovery behaviors accent and even magnify differences and incompatibilities. When everyone in the family has a recovery program, there is more room for a focus on interpersonal issues that does not threaten the stability of the individual's recovery.

The Coalcoholic in the Ongoing Recovery Stage

The process of Ongoing Recovery for the coalcoholic is identical to that of the alcoholic: a focus on the self with an opportunity for deeper exploration of past and present and an expansion in attention to include the partner in the couple relationship. With a foundation of recovery, the coalcoholic can focus on the couple without experiencing a loss of self, or a submission of self to an unhealthy dependence on the partner (Brown, 1988).

This process of maintaining separateness while joining together is the heart of healthy relationship. Because the coalcoholic has typically been obsessively focused on the alcoholic in the past, it is often tricky to know when the turn back to the partner is in the service of a healthy relationship and when it is not. Even with a clearer sense of self and a strong recovery, issues of intimacy and equal relationship bring up confusion, especially regarding boundaries and responsibility. The coalcoholic may experience fear that deeper intimacy will mean a relapse. The greater closeness almost certainly will raise initial confusion regarding detachment, engagement, and enmeshment. After several years of individual recovery Martina Torres (above) illustrates:

"I was angry at first. I didn't want to do this. I didn't want to have a part in it all. Why do I have to work on our relationship? I didn't want to drag Ryan along, which is how it felt. I wanted him to keep taking care of himself, and I would take care of me. We went to couples counseling, and I got excited. We were working on this together."

In order to learn the difference between healthy and unhealthy, the coalcoholic must pay continuing attention to his or her individual issues and program of recovery, just like the alcoholic. The opportunity for a healthy, close relationship is based on a foundation of being separate. Continuing to focus on oneself protects both partners from slipping back into old beliefs and patterns of behavior based on the need to control the partner.

Brenda Sandburg (above) talks about the process:

"I like myself a lot better. And we've become much closer. I learned to walk out and not participate. Before, I tried to make peace, to not ruffle the waters. In the first few years of recovery I was afraid. I was scared of what Russ would do to me and the kids. He was shutdown and full of anger. I used to comfort the kids when he would yell. I'd ask them not to say things, not to upset him. I've had to come to terms with all of this. . . . Then I got a voice. I got help and began to confront him and set my limits. It's been a long road looking at myself and becoming able to speak. The turning point came the first time I said no, I wouldn't go along with 'business as usual, minus alcohol.' I just couldn't do it anymore. In the last few years, I've felt heard and that is making all the difference. First I got me and now we are working on 'us.' "

Harold York shares his experience of 13 years in recovery:

"Over the years I have had to look at myself so closely. I started this marriage with a deep sense of inferiority and a driven need to achieve. I worked all the time and paid no attention to my wife and kids. Through many years of Al-Anon and a men's group, I have learned to shift my focus from work to relationship. At first, Abbie wasn't ready, but now we're much more involved with each other. I still watch out for my own issues. Abbie does a lot on her own, which can still throw me, as I have a lot of fears of abandonment. These childhood feelings come up, and I get scared. I've talked a great deal about my feelings in Al-Anon, and I talk with Abbie too. She doesn't necessarily change what she's doing, but we avoid tension between us. I don't take what she does as a personal attack on me, as I now recognize it often has nothing to do with me."

As Harold notes, childhood feelings and issues come up. They are bound to if recovery is going well. Martina Torres (above), with 8 years in Al-Anon and ACOA, has been coping with deep pain related to growing up with two severely alcoholic parents. Martina vividly recalls the frightening deaths of both of them, her father by suicide. When Ryan had several years of recovery, she felt secure enough to take her focus off of worrying about him and put in onto herself. Martina says that she has been dealing with the trauma of her life all her life but only in the last few years has she felt that she is really working some of it through as opposed to simply enduring it constantly. She now can see that her painful fears of what would happen to Ryan were a replay of her chronic childhood terror that her parents—drunk and often passed out—were dying:

"I have hurt so much in recovery. But it's been so much better. Ryan supports me to do this painful remembering and grieving because of all the help he got working through the trauma of Vietnam. I have faced so much I never thought would see the light of day."

The Children in the Ongoing Recovery Stage

If all goes well, each parent has developed a strong recovery program, having taken the time to focus on him- or herself early on. As a result, in Ongoing Recovery they both have more energy and ability to turn their attention to their children. They may be better able to hear and acknowledge feelings, and better able to deal directly with the past, taking responsibility and talking with their children about the realities of what happened during the drinking. Of course, the degree to which the realities of the past can be raised depends on the ages of the children, what happened, and the needs and capacities of the kids to hear and integrate the parents' stories. It is not helpful if the parents raise issues from the past in the service of their own needs when the child or ACOA cannot or does not want to hear these things. Hearing what a parent did and how a parent felt may be retraumatizing for a child.

A teenager tells us it was hard to hear parents talk about what they did. She doesn't remember feeling scared at the time, but it's scary now to hear it. Although the desire to tell about the past may stem from a parent's need more than the best interests of the child, the opposite can also be true. In many families, the recounting of reality, with parents telling their children exactly what happened, can be vitally important to healing. A therapist can help parents sort out what's important to reveal and what's not. It's especially important not to continue role reversal, with parents relying on children as confidants/confidantes and supporters of their recovery.

Secrets from the past can continue to exert a negative influence even though the family has many years of solid recovery. So it is extremely helpful if parents can respond honestly and openly to the children's request for information. We saw many families literally rewriting family history with their grown children. These adults needed to hear their parents tell the truth about all that happened during the drinking and during the early years of recovery for their own repair, integration, and healthy development. In one of our families, the children did not want to hear about the past until they were grown. Each child sought information about the drinking and all that happened after they were out of the home, pursuing their independent lives. Earlier, they had been too afraid of being drawn back into the family system.

In some of our families, grown children declined to participate in the interview because they did not want to hear about alcoholism or recovery. Several parents told us their children did not want their own denial of alcoholism and their still-idealized views of childhood disturbed, while others said that their children were so angry or (unfortunately) caught up in their own addiction that they had rejected the parents and recovery outright. In several families, grown children expressed their worry about their actively addicted siblings who were not present. One group of adult siblings told us they expected their older sister to die of alcoholism, as she has repeatedly refused their efforts to help her.

The reality of addicted children and/or the potential that children will become alcoholic is a part of all our research families' concerns. How they deal with it is likely to be a critical issue for all at some point. By Ongoing Recovery, each family has usually had to face the issue, if not solve it.

In several of our families, the children turned to alcohol and other drugs as soon as their parents entered recovery, so at first nothing changed. The environment remained chaotic and dominated by drinking, though it was now the children's active use and the parents' crisis of Transition that maintained it. When both parents stabilized in Early Recovery, they were able to address their children's problems differently. The environment became safer, reflecting their growing individual recoveries and their ability to be responsible parents. With help, they established an abstinent systems structure that would not incorporate active alcoholism. The alcoholism of the children became deviant in the system, whereas the alcoholism of the parents had been normative.

Many of our research families were second marriages, some with "blendings" of many children. Martina and Ryan Torres (above) share five children between them, none conceived together. Martina tells us how these grown kids differ in their experiences of their parents'/ steparents' recovery:

"Mitch, who has been close to both of us throughout, sees us as a normal couple. Leslie, who's in treatment for chemical dependence right now, is suspicious of what we have. She is angry and doesn't trust us. Nicole is happy we're in recovery and looks to us for support. Curt feels the same. He comes to talk with us often about himself and about life. He wants to see how we live and how we do it. And finally Wes—he's always lived [elsewhere] with his mother and violent, alcoholic stepfather. He thinks we're crazy when we have problems and talk about recovery. We look like the Cleavers compared to what he's grown up with."

This is a wonderful example of how much each child's experience depends on the individual's perspective and circumstances of the past and the present. When they were growing up, each of these children had a different experience of Martina and Ryan that they bring to their perceptions, beliefs, and experiences of Martina and Ryan in the present.

For most of the families who participated in our research, recovery is a family affair. By Ongoing Recovery, there is a long history—both of drinking and sobriety—to share. With many years of abstinence and growth in recovery, children reflect the positives of healthy change.

In the Hanson family, Burt, the eldest child, entered recovery 8 years prior to our meeting with them. His father stopped drinking and began recovery two years later and his mother had 13 months of abstinence. Burt tells us that he had been through two recoveries: his own and his family's:

> "I learned a lot about myself in the beginning, particularly how to detach from all of them to protect myself. They were still drinking. But after Dad got sober, things changed a lot. We spent years with a split in our world: we talked recovery and got a lot closer while Mom kept drinking. But the family became 'recovering' anyway. Now that Mom is also sober, everything is different. I've changed my view of myself a lot in the last year as we talk so much more from the same perspective. Now, we have a family story that we mostly agree on."

Burt illustrates the importance of the recovery lens, which colors everything. Recall that this lens is centered on an acceptance of loss of control, while the still-drinking individual has a vested interest in maintaining a belief in control. The therapist working with the Hanson family 15 months ago repeatedly pointed out the reality of different beliefs and how hard it was to have family unity as a result. Now, the family is engaged as a whole, reflected in a family story they are constructing together.

Luke Hanson, the second son, expands on the benefits of his mother's recovery:

> "I have taken a lot from her example. She is somebody I can learn from now because she's modeling healthy behavior and attitudes. Her reactions to things are more thought out, more logical, and things make sense. I could never rely on her before. Now I am more rational and responsible as a result of seeing her change."

Younger children may have less need for repair as they continue their normal development with sober parents. In Ongoing Recovery there is greater freedom to focus on appropriate child or adolescent developmental issues, such as the freedom to talk and disagree with parents, to leave the family at age-appropriate times, or to have friends over without fear or embarrassment. Improvements in the parents' relationship provide greater safety for children to test limits with the trust that boundaries will be held, parent–child roles maintained, and protection ensured.

Parents can deal with crises now in healthier ways. They maintain their own sobriety and preserve the safety and security of the family system. One coalcoholic parent tells us she remained calm when her son was recently injured on the playing field. "This was a big change," she says. "Before, I would have been too hysterical to help my son, or comfort him. He would have had to take care of *me*."

The inner sense of stability and trust that comes with Ongoing Recovery holds everybody in the family through difficult times. If only one parent is in recovery and there is conflict between the parents about recovery, children will continue to have trouble focusing on their own development. Some of our research families report that having parents at different stages of recovery was also difficult, adding to an anxious environment and systems problems similar to the drinking times.

For most families, Ongoing Recovery offers the healthiest environment, family system, and parents yet possible. The parents' strong individual development, their adherence to values of honesty and integrity, and their new capacity to function as a healthy couple offer their children a second chance.

Epilogue

In the summer of 1998, just before our manuscript was sent to the typesetter, we wrote to our research participants, informing them about the completion of this book and requesting their permission to quote them directly. We heard from over 70% of our sample and talked with many of them by phone.

Most of the people who responded, and all of the 28 couples with whom we spoke, told us they are still sober and that their lives are richer, fuller, and more satisfying than they had been at the time of their interview, which occurred from 5 to 7 years earlier. Thus, many of our research families have moved from Transition or Early Recovery to Ongoing Recovery. One family, who had 5 years of recovery in 1991, now has 12. Another, who had 12 years when we met them, now has 19 and all the kids are grown. One of our last families had 4 years at the time of the interview; they happily reported 8 years now. Some wrote us notes, with an update on children, many of whom are still in recovery themselves or have entered recovery for their own addictions. In some cases, we learned that grown children are currently struggling with alcohol and other drug problems and relationship issues.

Many people affirmed the ongoing importance to them of AA and Al-Anon and credited these programs for their continuing abstinence and successful recoveries. Several participants told us they have become active in Al-Anon since the interview, and several reported that their children also participate in a 12-step program.

Sadly, one of our subjects, Tony Castle, died of natural causes. His wife, Denise, said he had achieved 14 years of very satisfying, fulfilling sobriety. She continues to attend Al-Anon regularly, adding that she enjoys giving to others what was given to her. She also said that "our recovery improved greatly over the years."

Josh Corwin told us he celebrated 5 years of sobriety during the summer of 1998. He remembered the interview and the atmosphere of tension and anger we felt so acutely. Josh recalled that he was getting ready to drink, which he proceeded to do a few weeks after our meeting.

And one family, who had been in tremendous turmoil at the time of the interview, wrote that everyone is sober, and "even the dog is more relaxed."

Clearly, the majority of our sample are still sober, still identifying themselves in recovery from alcoholism, and still together as a couple.

We were touched by, and immensely grateful to, all our participants at the time of the interviews. We feel the same way now. Our research families gave us, then and now, astounding testimony to the power of sobriety and recovery.

Glossary

Abstinence: the state of not drinking alcohol or "using" any other addictive or intoxicating substances.

Alcoholic: a person who has lost behavioral and/or emotional control of his or her drinking.

Alcoholic thinking: denial, the "logic" that rationalizes drinking behavior and the necessity of drinking in a way that makes it plausible and maintains the behavior.

Alcoholism: a physical, psychological, social, emotional, and spiritual disorder/disease, characterized by continuous or periodic loss of control over drinking, preoccupation with the drug alcohol, use of alcohol despite adverse consequences, and distortions in thinking, most notably denial.

Boundaries: limits set by the individual, couple, and/or family: a family boundary is the imaginary line drawn around the family group; boundaries have permeable levels (allow entry and exit with ease or difficulty).

Change: an alteration that can occur over time (the life cycle) or in relation to a specific situation or crisis.

Coalcoholism: a compulsive preoccupation with controlling the alcoholic; the individual cannot focus on the self.

Codependence: follows from coalcoholism: any reactive, submissive response to the dominance of another; the individual sacrifices personal autonomy and choice to the control or perceived control of another.

Crisis: an emotionally significant event or radical change of status in a person's life; a decisive moment or turning point; any force that causes a system to destabilize from an old way of functioning.

Defense: unconscious behavior or thought process used by the individual, couple, and/or family to protect against painful or anxiety-provoking reality, including behavior, thought, or affect.

Denial: defense mechanism in which the individual cannot or will not acknowledge reality.

Development: a process of growth with specific and expected tasks and stages.

Domain: a distinctly delimited sphere of knowledge.

Dry: the state of abstinence: drinking is "wet"; not drinking is "dry."

Dry drunk: a state or condition in which an individual is not drinking (dry), yet experiences the same behavior, thinking, attitudes, and emotional reactions that characterize his or her active drinking.

Dynamic: pattern of forces in individual and family development.

Environment: the surrounding conditions and context of life; what an individual sees, hears, touches, tastes, and feels.

Family personality/family identity: a family's characteristic thinking style, belief system, values, temperament, cohesion, and emotional style (Reiss, 1981).

Hierarchy: the various subsystems of a family so ranked that one subsystem has higher authority than others (e.g., mother/father has authority over daughter/son).

Homeostasis: a point of internal balance.

Identity: fundamental core beliefs and sense of self.

Pathology: something abnormal: beliefs, traits, behaviors, defenses, or affects of an individual, couple, and/or family that contribute to, cause, and/or maintain problems.

Process: communication and interaction patterns: the action of passing through continuing development; a natural, progressively continuing operation.

Rationalization: a superficially plausible explanation or excuse.

Recovery: a multistage, multidomain developmental process in which the alcoholic, coalcoholic, and family move from drinking to maintaining abstinence.

Relapse: a return to the behaviors and thinking of drinking or using other drugs for the alcoholic; for the coalcoholic and family, a return to compulsive, controlling behavior, thinking, and affect in relation to the alcoholic.

Ritual: any behavior carried out in a prescribed way (e.g., a custom).

Role: a prescribed and repetitive behavior that involves interactions with others.

Rule: an accepted procedure, custom, or habit having the force of a regulation; may be explicit (directly communicated) or implicit (indirectly communicated).

Sobriety: the quality of the state of abstinence: one can be "dry" without being "sober"; one cannot be "sober" without also being "dry."

Spiritual: of or related to the moral feelings or states of a person's inner life, or soul, as distinguished from the external actions.

Stability: a condition in which a system is consistent, balanced, reliable, and predictable (related to homeostasis).

Stages: levels, periods, or phases in a process of development, growth, or change.

Step: a stage in a gradual, regular, or orderly process.

Structure: something having a definite or fixed pattern of organization; also, the way in which its parts are put together or organized; its form.

System: the relation of parts to a whole; a group whose components interact together in a consistent fashion.

Trauma: "the overwhelming of the self's normal preservative functioning in the face of inevitable danger" (Krystal, 1978).

Appendices

Throughout the text, we refer to the research sample, our 52 couples and families whose experiences of drinking and recovery formed the core principles of the developmental model of family recovery. In Appendix A we present the questionnaire that guided our semistructured research interviews. In Appendix B we summarize the significant characteristics of our sample, including numbers of alcoholics, coalcoholics, males, females, and length of sobriety. We also include a breakdown by age, years of drinking, history of parental or familial alcoholism, and membership in 12-step programs or other sources of support. These variables helped us determine similarities and differences in the sample subjects, and thus to more clearly delineate the stages and tasks in the developmental model.

As we mentioned in the preface, all our subjects were heterosexual couples. In addition, they had to have been together as an established couple for at least 5 years of active drinking, and they needed to be intact as a couple in recovery. With this before-and-after history, we could assess changes in the environment, in the structure and process of the family system, and within the individuals.

After we began the research and had difficulty finding subjects, we speculated that many, and perhaps even most, couples do not survive the drinking intact, or they do not survive 5 years of recovery.

We grouped families by length of abstinence. Yet we knew from prior research (Brown, 1985) that the tasks of development were more important in determining stage. We also found many other variables that contribute to stage and quality of recovery, which we have described throughout the text.

APPENDIX A. INTERVIEW QUESTIONS

1. What was it like for each of you during the drinking years? Please describe.

2. What was it like for you and your family when you started toward abstinence? Describe the turning points.
   a. Did you "hit bottom" or experience a surrender?
   b. What factors entered into "hitting bottom"?
   c. Were there critical events leading to abstinence?
      (1) Who made the decision to stop drinking?
      (2) Were children part of the decision making? What were they told?
   d. What adjustments did you and your family have to make? How easy or difficult were these adjustments? Who had the most difficult time?
   e. What was it like moving from drinking to recovery from each family member's point of view?
   f. How did you function in this transition period as a family? How did daily activities/ tasks get done? Who did them?
   g. How do you think your spouse saw the transition period (i.e., is the spouse in agreement)?
   h. Have you discussed this issue or thoughts and feelings related to it before?
   i. At the beginning, how did you feel about your partner going to AA meetings? Al-Anon?
   j. Who was most influential in your decision to stop drinking? How?

3. Do you see yourselves as an alcoholic family now? What does this mean to you?
   a. How did you get there? When? Does everyone agree that you are an alcoholic family? Was it always this way?
   b. What is it like? And how does it feel? Positive? Negative?
   c. Has your family been important to you in your recovery? If so, how? If not, why not?

4. How do you currently see your family dealing with life's crises, surprises, the unpredictable?
   a. How did the family deal with the period of change from drinking into recovery? How about dealing with the unexpected then and now?
   b. Do you see yourself and/or your family changing with time in how effective you are with these situations?
   c. What were the crises/difficulties then and now?

5. How has the decision process changed for you as a family from the beginning of abstinence to now?
   a. Who made decisions during active drinking, who made them during the move into recovery, and who makes them now?

b. Describe the process of decision making (e.g., we all talk about the concern, or one person decides and tells others, etc.).

6. How confident is the family now about sobriety? Has your level of confidence changed since the beginning? Does anybody worry?
   a. As a family, do you have a "program" or a ritual of recovery? As individuals, do you have a "program" of recovery? What is it?
   b. How does the family program help maintain the family's recovery? The individual's?
   c. Do you have an agreed-upon plan or strategy to deal with problems that arise in recovery?

7. How much is recovery a part of the family's life?
   a. AA programs—who attends, frequency, type? Is there a difference in attendance since the beginning of abstinence?
   b. As a whole, do you define yourselves as a recovering alcoholic family?
      (1) If yes, why?
      (2) If no, why?
   c. How central are the issues of alcoholism and recovery to the family as a whole and individually?

8. Has it felt to you that there have been stages in your process of recovery as a family? As individuals? What are they?
   a. Can anybody remember when the beginning of the end started? That is, when did the move into recovery begin? Who made the first move? What was the impact? How and why have others in the family joined in recovery?
   b. Was there a time or event when you saw yourselves clearly grounded in family recovery? When? What?

9. Recovery over time:
   a. What's it been like for the family? For the individuals? (From very comfortable to very uncomfortable—why?)
   b. What major adjustments has the family had to make since the beginning of abstinence?
   c. What major issues other than alcoholism has the family had to deal with in recovery?
   d. Who has been the most meaningful person to each of you in the recovery process? Does anybody stand out as most important to the family as a whole?
   e. Can you imagine what it would be like if you were not now a recovering family?
   f. What does the family think of this statement: alcoholism is a progressive illness; recovery is also a progressive process?
   g. Do you think there is such a thing as "backward steps" in recovery? If so, describe them.

   h. How about problems in recovery?
- (1) Who recognized them in the family early on? Who recognizes them now? How long did/does it take to recognize, name, and deal with difficulties?
- (2) Have there been "slips" or relapses in this family, and how have you dealt with them?

   i. What is the family doing to maintain recovery? Specific details.

10. Family "story":
   a. As a family do you have a shared story about your recovery?
   b. Have you ever talked together about the drinking and recovery process? Ever thought about the idea of a family story, or a family "drunkalogue"?
   c. How has the history of alcoholism in the family been compiled? Who's in charge of the history, or family story? Does everyone contribute? Does each person now have an individual story about drinking and recovery as well?

APPENDIX B. RESULTS OF THE FAMILY RECOVERY RESEARCH PROJECT

TABLE B.1. Demographics

Variables	Numbers (%)
Couples	52
Alcoholics	
Women	23 (39.0%)
Men	36 (61.0%)
Age (years)	
Range	28–69
Mean	48.31 (SD = 9.71)
Marital status	
First marriage	53 (51%)
Second or more marriages	42 (40.4%)
Partners	4 (3.8%)
(missing 4.8%)	
Children	
With children	84 (80.8%)
Without children	16 (15.4%)
(missing 3.8%)	
Ethnicity	
Caucasians	97 (93.3%)
Hispanics	3 (2.9%)
(missing 3.8%)	
Highest degree	
None	3 (2.9%)
High school	30 (28.8%)
AA (associate in arts) degree	13 (12.5%)
College	24 (23.1%)
Graduate training	29 (27.9%)
(missing 4.8%)	
Occupation level	
Professional/executive positions	52 (50.0%)
Administrative/clerical	18 (17.3%)
Education	7 (6.7%)
Skilled manual positions	4 (3.8%)
Homemakers and students	17 (16.3%)
Unemployed	1 (1.0%)
(missing 4.8%)	
Income level	
$16,000–40,000	17 (17.3%)
$41,000–75,000	38 (36.5%)
$76,000–150,000	34 (32.7%)
Over $150,000	6 (5.8%)
(missing 7.7%)	
Program (currently)	86.4% of alcoholics, 53.3% of coalcoholics
AA	84.2% of alcoholics, 4.4% of coalcoholics
Al-Anon	5.3% of alcoholics, 48.9% of coalcoholics

TABLE B.2. Numbers of Alcoholics and Coalcoholics

	Coalcoholic		Alcoholic	
	Count	Col %	Count	Col %
Female	30	66.7%	23	39.0%
Male	15	33.3%	36	61.0%

Note. Coalcoholics: 66.7% female, 33.3% male; alcoholics: 39% female, 61% male.

TABLE B.3. Length of Recovery for Alcoholics

Valid	Frequency	%
0 to 12 months	10	16.9
1+ years to 3 years	12	20.3
3+ years to 5 years	10	16.9
5+ years to 10 years	19	32.2
10+ years	8	13.6
Total	59	100.0

Note. Mean number of months in recovery: 62.31; minimum: 2 months; maximum: 215 months (17.9 years).

TABLE B.4a. Alcoholics and Coalcoholics Who Had Alcoholic Parent(s)

	Nonalcoholic		Alcoholic	
Parent(s) alcoholic	Count	Col %	Count	Col %
Yes	19	44.2%	34	60.7%
No	24	55.8%	22	39.3%

Note. 60.7% of alcoholics had an alcoholic parent; 44.2% of coalcoholics had an alcoholic parent.

TABLE B.4b. All Subjects by Alcoholic Parent(s)

		Frequency	%
Valid	Yes	53	51.0
	No	46	44.2
	Total	99	95.2
Missing	System missing	5	4.8
	Total	5	4.8
Total		104	100.0

Note. A similar number of subjects with and without alcoholic parent(s) (51% vs. 44.2%).

TABLE B.5a. Psychotherapy before Recovery: All Subjects

		Frequency	%
Valid	Yes	59	56.7
	No	38	36.5
	Total	97	93.3
Missing	System missing	7	6.7
	Total	7	6.7
Total		104	100.0

Note. 56.7% of all subjects had some psychotherapy before sobriety began; 36.5% did not have any psychotherapy before.

TABLE B.5b. Psychotherapy before Recovery: Alcoholics versus Coalcoholics

Psychotherapy before recovery	Nonalcoholic		Alcoholic	
	Count	Col %	Count	Col %
Yes	22	52.4%	37	67.3%
No	20	47.6%	18	32.7%

Note. There was no significant difference in the numbers of alcoholics and coalcoholics who had/did not have therapy before sobriety began.

TABLE B.6a. Psychotherapy after Recovery: All Subjects

		Frequency	%
Valid	Yes	53	51.0
	No	46	44.2
	Total	99	95.2
Missing	System missing	5	4.8
	Total	5	4.8
Total		104	100.0

Note. 51% of all subjects (53) participated in psychotherapy after recovery began; 44.2% of all subjects (46) did not participate in psychotherapy.

TABLE B.6b. Psychotherapy after Recovery: Alcoholics versus Coalcoholics

Psychotherapy after recovery	Nonalcoholic		Alcoholic	
	Count	Col %	Count	Col %
Yes	21	48.8%	32	57.1%
No	22	51.2%	24	42.9%

Note. Alcoholics and coalcoholics were similar in participation rate in therapy postsobriety (57.1% vs. 48.8%).

TABLE B.7. Children

Total of children: 84

Total of children participated in study: 41

TABLE B.8. Marital Composition

For first marriage 52 (51%) of subjects were married only that one time.

For second marriage or more, 42 subjects (40.4%) were married more than once.

There were no significant differences between alcoholics and coalcoholics and no significant difference between men and women in these percentages.

TABLE B.9. Alcoholics and Coalcoholics' Parents in Recovery

Valid	Frequency	%	Valid %	Cumulative %
Yes	4	5.7	5.7	5.7
No	66	94.3	94.3	100.0
Total	70	100.0	100.0	

Note. 5.7% of parents of our subjects (alcoholics and coalcoholics) were in recovery; 94.3% were not in recovery.

TABLE B.10. Recreational Activities for Couples: Alcoholics and Coalcoholics

Attending parties: 28% never/rarely attend, 43.3% sometimes attend, 23% attend frequently/often.

Working on hobbies: 14.4% rarely work, 32.7% sometimes work, 47% work frequently on hobbies.

Attending church: 55% never/rarely attend, 11.5% sometimes attend, 27% attend frequently/often.

Attending social club: 57% never/rarely attend, 27% sometimes attend, 10% attend frequently/often.

Meeting with friends: 6.7% rarely meet with friends, 26% sometimes meet, 52% meet with friends frequently/often.

Designated time with family: 12.5% rarely have time with family, 28.8% sometimes, 53% have frequently/often designated time with family.

Community activities: 34% rarely/never participate, 45.2% participate sometimes, 15% participate in community activities frequently/often.

Playing sports: 46% never/rarely play, 23.1% sometimes play, 16% frequently/often play sports.

Watching TV: 6% never/rarely watch TV, 17.3% sometimes watch TV, 71% frequently/often watch TV.

Reading: 2.9% rarely read, 16.3% sometimes read, 76% read frequently/often.

Attending cultural events: 31% rarely attend, 45.2% sometimes attend, 17% frequently/often attend cultural events.

Watching movies: 21.2% rarely watch, 26.9% sometimes watch, 46% frequently/often watch movies.

Attending sports events: 52% rarely/never attend, 32.7% sometimes attend, 10% frequently/often attend sports events.

TABLE B.11. Frequency of Current Attendance at AA/Al-Anon: Alcoholics versus Coalcoholics

		None	Once every few months	Once every few weeks	Once a week	2–4 times a week	5 or more times a week
Coalcoholic	Count	22	6	6	6	4	—
	Col %	50.0%	13.6%	13.6%	13.6%	9.1%	—
Alcoholic	Count	7	9	4	8	23	5
	Col %	12.5%	16.1%	7.1%	14.3%	41.1%	8.9%

Note. In current participation there were differences between alcoholics and coalcoholics in program attendance patterns. The frequency patterns are very noticeable at the extreme points. Under "None" (no attendance) there are 50% of coalcoholics versus only 12.5% alcoholics. Under the category "2–4 times a week" there are 41.1% of alcoholics versus 9.1% of coalcoholics.

TABLE B.12. Frequency of Current Attendance at AA/Al-Anon: All Subjects

	Valid								
	None	Once every few months	Once every few weeks	Once a week	2–4 times a week	5 or more times a week	Total	Missing	Total
Frequency	29	15	10	14	27	5	100	4	104
%	27.9	14.4	9.6	13.5	26.0	4.8	96.2	3.8	100.0

Note. Participation ranged from none (27.9%) to some level of attendance (68.3%), with the greater attendance in the "2–4 times a week" category (26%).

TABLE B.13. Years Alcohol Has Been a Problem (for Alcoholics)

		Frequency	%
Valid	1–2 years	1	1.7
	2–5 years	7	11.9
	5–10 years	11	18.6
	10–15 years	19	32.2
	15+ years	17	28.8
	Total	55	93.2
Missing	System missing	4	6.8
	Total	4	6.8
Total		59	100.0

Note. How long alcohol has been a problem for alcoholics before recovery by frequency: 1–2 years (2%); 2–5 years (12%); 5–10 years (19%); 10–15 years (32%); and 15+ (29%); missing (7%).

TABLE B.14. Gender by Depression since Sobriety: Alcoholics

	Depression since sobriety in family		
	Yes	No	Total
Female	18	4	22
Male	12	20	32
Total	30	24	54

Note. There were 18 women alcoholics and 12 men alcoholics who experienced depression. On no depression there is a *significant difference* between men and women. Only 4 women versus 20 men who experienced no depression.

TABLE B.15. Depression since Sobriety by Alcoholism: All Subjects

	Depression since sobriety in family		
	Yes	No	Total
Nonalcoholic	18	25	43
Alcoholic	30	24	54
Total	48	29	97

Note. There was no *significant difference* proportionately between alcoholics and coalcoholics on depression or no depression since sobriety.

TABLE B.16. Subjects Who Felt Suicidal in Recovery by Alcoholism

	Felt suicidal in recovery		
	Yes	No	Total
Nonalcoholic	2	41	43
Alcoholic	18	35	53
Total	20	76	96

Note. There was a significant difference between alcoholic and coalcoholic groups on feeling suicidal since sobriety. Only 2 (out of 43) coalcoholics felt suicidal versus 18 (out of 53) alcoholics who felt suicidal.

TABLE B.17. Age of Recovery for Alcoholics

	Age group	Frequency	%
Valid	20–25	1	1.7
	25–30	5	8.5
	30–35	11	18.6
	35–40	7	11.9
	40–45	19	16.9
	45–50	10	16.9
	50+	12	20.3
	Total	56	94.9
Missing	System missing	3	5.1
	Total	3	5.1
Total		59	100.0

Note. Most alcoholics studied began recovery between 30 and 50 years of age (64.3%). Frequency in age groups: 20–26 years (1.7%); 25–30 years (8.5%); 30–35 years (18.6%); 35–40 years (11.9%); 40–45 years (16.9%); 45–50 years (16.9%); and 50+ (20.3%).

References

Ackerman, N., Papp, P., & Prosky, P. Childhood disorders and interlocking pathology in family relationships. In E. J. Anthony & C. Koupernick (Eds.), *The Child in His Family: Children at Psychiatric Risk*. New York: Wiley-Interscience, 1970, pp. 241–266.

Ackerman, N. Toward an integrative therapy of the family. *American Journal of Psychiatry, 114*, 1958, 727–733.

Ackerman, N. *The Psychodynamics of Family Life: Diagnosis and Treatment of Family Relationships*. Northvale, NJ: Aronson, 1994.

Al-Anon Faces Alcoholism. New York: Al-Anon Family Groups, 1984.

Alcoholics Anonymous. *Twelve Steps and Twelve Traditions*. New York: Alcoholics Anonymous World Services, 1952.

Alcoholics Anonymous. New York: AA World Services, 1955.

Amodeo, M. A. The therapist's role in the drinking stage. In S. Brown (Ed.), *Treating Alcoholism*. San Francisco: Jossey-Bass, 1995a, pp. 95–132.

Amodeo, M. A. The therapist's role in the transition stage. In S. Brown (Ed.), *Treating Alcoholism*. San Francisco: Jossey-Bass, 1995b, pp. 133–162.

Bader, E., & Pearson, P. *In Quest of the Mythical Mate: A Developmental Approach to Diagnosis and Treatment in Couples Therapy*. New York: Brunner/Mazel, 1988.

Bateson, G. The cybernetics of self: A theory of alcoholism. *Psychiatry, 34*(1), 1971, 1–18.

Bean, M. Alcoholics Anonymous I. *Psychiatric Annals, 5*(2), 1975a, 7–61.

Bean, M. Alcoholics Anonymous II. *Psychiatric Annals, 5*(3), 1975b, 7–57.

Bean, M. Denial and the psychological complications of alcoholism. In M. Bean & N. Zinberg (Eds.), *Dynamic Approaches to the Understanding and Treatment of Alcoholism*. New York: Free Press, 1981, pp. 55–96.

Bean-Bayog, M. Psychopathology produced by alcoholism. In R. E. Meyer (Ed.), *Psychopathology and Addictive Disorders*. New York: Guilford Press, 1986, pp. 334–345.

Berger, P. & Luckman, T. *The Social Construction of Reality*. New York: Anchor Books, 1966.

Black, C. *It Will Never Happen to Me*. Denver: MAC, 1981.

Blos, P., *On Adolescence: A Psychoanalytic Interpretation*. New York: Free Press, 1962.

Bowen, M. Alcoholism as viewed through family systems theory and psychother-apy. *Annals of the New York Academy of Science, 233*, 1974, 115–122.

Bowen, M. *Family Therapy in Clinical Practice*. Northvale, NJ: Aronson, 1978.

Bowlby, J. *Attachment and Loss* (Vol. 3). New York: Basic Books, 1980.

Bowlby, J. The role of childhood experience in cognitive disturbance. In M. Mahoney & A. Freeman (Eds.), *Cognition and Psychotherapy*. New York: Plenum, 1985, pp. 181–200.

Bowlby, J. *A Secure Base*. New York: Basic Books, 1988.

Brown, S. *Defining a Process of Recovery in Alcoholism*. Doctoral Dissertation, California School of Professional Psychology, Berkeley, 1977.

Brown, S. *Treating the Alcoholic: A Developmental Model of Recovery*. New York: Wiley, 1985.

Brown, S. Children with an alcoholic parent. In N. J. Estes & M. E. Heinemann (Eds.), *Alcoholism: Development, Consequences and Interventions*. St. Louis, MO: Mosby, 1986, pp. 207–220.

Brown, S. *Treating Adult Children of Alcoholics: A Developmental Perspective*. New York: Wiley, 1988.

Brown, S. Adult children of alcoholics: The history of a social movement and its impact on clinical theory and practice. In M. Galanter (Ed.), *Recent Developments in Alcoholism* (Vol. 9). New York: Plenum, 1991a, pp. 267–285.

Brown, S. Children of chemically dependent parents: A theoretical crossroads. In T. Rivinus (Ed.), *Children of Chemically Dependent Parents: Multiperspec-tives from the Cutting Edge*. New York: Brunner/Mazel, 1991b, pp. 74–102.

Brown, S. *Safe Passage: Recovery for Adult Children of Alcoholics*. New York: Wiley, 1991c.

Brown, S. Therapeutic processes in Alcoholics Anonymous. In B. McCrady & W. Miller (Eds.), *Research on Alcoholics Anonymous*. New Brunswick, NJ: Rutgers Center of Alcohol Studies, 1993, pp. 137–152.

Brown, S. Alcoholism and trauma: A theoretical comparison and overview. *Journal of Psychoactive Drugs, 26*(4), 1994, 345–355.

Brown, S. A developmental model of alcoholism and recovery. In S. Brown (Ed.), *Treating Alcoholism*. San Francisco: Jossey-Bass, 1995a, pp. 27–53.

Brown, S. (Ed.). *Treating Alcoholism*. San Francisco: Jossey-Bass, 1995b.

Brown, S. Adult children of alcoholics: An expanded framework for assessment and diagnosis. In S. Abbott (Ed.), *Children of Alcoholics: Selected Readings*. Rockville, MD: National Association for Children of Alcoholics, 1995c, pp. 41–76.

Brown, S., Beletsis, S., & Cermak, T. *Adult Children of Alcoholics in Treatment*. Orlando, FL: Health Communications, 1989.

Brown, S., & Lewis, V. The alcoholic family: A developmental model of recovery. In S. Brown (Ed.) *Treating Alcoholism*. San Francisco: Jossey-Bass, 1995, pp. 279–315.

Butcher, J. N., Dahlstrom, W. G., Graham, J. R., Tellegen, A. M. & Kaemmer, B. *MMPI II: Manual for Administration and Scoring*. Minneapolis, MN: University of Minnesota Press, 1989.

Cannon, W. *The Wisdom of the Body.* New York: Norton, 1932.

Cermak, T. *Diagnosing and Treating Codependence.* Minneapolis MN: The Johnson Institute, 1986.

Dorpat, T. *Denial and Defense in the Therapeutic Situation.* New York: Aronson, 1985.

Erikson, E. *Childhood and Society.* New York: Norton, 1963.

Eth, S., & Pynoos, R. *Post-Traumatic Stress Disorder in Children.* Washington, DC: American Psychiatric Press, 1985.

Flavell, J. *The Developmental Psychology of Jean Piaget.* Princeton, NJ: Van Nostrand, 1963.

Fowler, J. Alcoholics Anonymous and faith development. In B. McCrady & W. Miller (Eds.), *Research on Alcoholics Anonymous.* New Brunswick, NJ: Rutgers Center of Alcohol Studies, 1993, pp. 113–135.

Goleman, D. *Vital Lies and Simple Truths.* New York: Simon & Schuster, 1985.

Gorski, T. The Cenaps model of relapse prevention: Basic principles and procedures. *Journal of Psychoactive Drugs,* 22(2), 1990, 125–133.

Greenspan, S. I. *Intelligence and Adaptation: An Integration of Psychoanalytic and Piagetian Developmental Psychology.* New York: International Universities Press, 1979.

Guidano, V., & Liotti, G. *Cognitive Processes and Emotional Disorders.* New York: Guilford Press, 1983.

Guntrip, H. *Schizoid Problems, Object-Relations, and the Self.* New York: International Universities Press, 1968.

Gurman, A., & Kniskern, D. (Eds.). *Handbook of Family Therapy.* New York: Brunner/Mazel, 1981.

Haley, J. *Uncommon Therapy: The Psychiatric Techniques of Milton Erickson.* New York: Norton, 1973.

Hartocollis, P. A dynamic view of alcoholism: Drinking in the service of denial. *Dynamic Psychiatry,* 6, 1968, 309–325.

Hartocollis, P., & Hartocollis, P. Alcoholism, borderline, and narcissistic disorders: A psychoanalytic overview. In E. Farr, I. Haracan, A. Pokorny, & R. Williams (Eds.), *Phenomenology and Treatment of Alcoholism.* New York: SP Medical & Scientific Books, 1980, pp. 893–1110.

Heimannsberg, B. & Schmidt, C. (Eds.). *The Collective Silence: German Identity and the Legacy of Shame.* San Francisco: Jossey-Bass, 1993.

Herman, J. *Trauma and Recovery.* New York: Basic Books, 1992.

Jackson, J. The adjustment of the family to the crisis of alcoholism. *Quarterly Journal of Studies on Alcohol,* 15, 1954, 562–586.

Jackson, J. Alcoholism and the family. In D. J. Pittman & C. R. Snyder (Eds.), *Society, Culture and Drinking Patterns.* New York: Wiley, 1962.

Jacob, T. (Ed.). *Family Interaction and Psychotherapy: Theories, Methods and Findings.* New York: Plenum, 1987.

Jacob, T., Favorini, A., Meisel, S. S., & Anderson, C. M. The alcoholic's spouse, children and family interactions: Substantive findings and methodological issues. *Journal of Studies on Alcohol,* 38, 1978, 1231–1251.

Jacob, T., Dunn, J. N., & Leonard, K. Patterns of alcohol abuse and family stability. *Alcoholism: Clinical and Experimental Research,* 7, 1981, 382–385.

Jellinek, E. M. *The Disease Concept of Alcoholism.* New Haven, CT: College & University Press, 1960.

Kagan, J. *The Nature of the Child*. New York: Basic Books, 1984.

Katz, R. & Ney, N., Preventing relapse. In S. Brown (Ed.), *Treating Alcoholism*. San Francisco: Jossey-Bass, 1995, 231–276.

Kaufman, E. *Psychotherapy of Addicted Persons*. New York: Guilford Press, 1994.

Khan, M. M. R., The concept of cumulative trauma. *Psychoanalytic Study of the Child*, 18, 1963, 286–306.

Khantzian, E. J. Some treatment implications of ego and self-disturbances in alcoholism. In M. Bean & N. Zinberg (Eds.), *Dynamic Approaches to the Understanding and Treatment of Alcoholism*. New York: Free Press, 1981, pp. 163–188.

Khantzian, E. J., Halliday, K. S., & McAuliffe, W. E. *Addiction and the Vulnerable Self*. New York: Guilford Press, 1990.

Krugman, S. Trauma in the family: Perspectives on the intergenerational transmission of violence. In B. van der Kolk (Ed.), *Psychological Trauma*. Washington, DC: American Psychiatric Press, 1987, pp. 127–152.

Krystal, H. Trauma and affects. *Psychoanalytic Study of the Child*, 33, 1978, 127–152.

Krystal, H., & Raskin, H. *Drug Dependence: Aspects of Ego Function*. Northvale, NJ: Aronson, 1993.

Levin, J. *Treatment of Alcoholism and Other Addictions: A Self-Psychology Approach*. Northvale, NJ: Aronson, 1987.

Levin, J. *Couple and Family Therapy of Addiction*. Northvale, NJ: Aronson, 1998.

Lewis, V. *The Family Recovery Typology Model*. Unpublished manuscript, The Family Recovery Project, Mental Research Institute, Palo Alto, CA, 1997.

Lewis, V., & Atzmon, O. *MMPI Data*. Unpublished manuscript. The Family Recovery Project, Mental Research Institute, Palo Alto, CA, 1997.

Liftik, J. Assessment. In S. Brown (Ed.), *Treating Alcoholism*. San Francisco: Jossey-Bass, 1995, pp. 57–93.

Lifton, R. *Nazi Doctors*. New York: Basic Books, 1986.

Mahler, M., Pine, T., & Bergman, H. *The Psychological Birth of the Human Infant*. New York: Basic Books, 1975.

Mahoney, M. Psychotherapy and human change processes. In M. Mahoney & A. Freeman (Eds.), *Cognition and Psychotherapy*. New York: Plenum, 1985, pp. 3–48.

Mahoney, M. The cognitive sciences and psychotherapy: Patterns in a developing relationship. In K. S. Dobson (Ed.), *Handbook of Cognitive-Behavioral Therapies*. New York: Guilford Press, 1988, pp. 357–386.

Marlatt, G. A. The controlled drinking controversy: A commentary. *American Psychologist*, 38(10), 1983, 1097–1110.

Marlatt, G. A., & Gordon, J. R. (Eds.). *Relapse Prevention: Maintenance Strategies in the Treatment of Addictive Behaviors*. New York: Guilford Press, 1985.

Minuchin, S. Constructing a therapeutic reality. In E. Kaufman & P. Kaufman (Eds.), *Family Therapy of Drug and Alcohol Abuse* (2nd ed.). Boston: Allyn & Bacon, 1992, pp. 1–14.

Minuchin, S., & Fishman, C. *Family Therapy Techniques*. Cambridge, MA: Harvard University Press, 1981.

Minuchin, S., Montalvo, B., Guerney, B., Rosman, B., & Schumer, F. *Families of the Slums: An Exploration of Their Structure and Treatment*. New York: Basic Books, 1967.

Moe, J. Small steps becoming large: Effective strategies to assist children of alcoholics in the healing process. In S. Abbott (Ed.), *Children of Alcoholics: Selected Readings*. Rockville, MD: National Association for Children of Alcoholics, 1995, pp. 137–152.

Nace, E. The dual diagnosis patient. In S. Brown (Ed.), *Treating Alcoholism*. San Francisco: Jossey-Bass, 1995, pp. 163–193.

Ogden, T. *The Matrix of the Mind*. New York: Aronson, 1986.

Ogden, T. *The Primitive Edge of Experience*. New York: Aronson, 1989.

Pendery, M., Maltzman, I., & West, L. J. Controlled drinking by alcoholics?: New findings and a reevaluation of a major affirmative study. *Science, 217,* 1982, 169–174.

Piaget, J. *The Construction of Reality in the Child*. New York: Basic Books, 1954.

Piaget, J. Piaget's theory. In P. Mussen (Ed.), *Carmichael's Manual of Child Psychology* (3rd ed.). New York: Wiley, 1970.

Reiss, D. *The Family's Construction of Reality*. Cambridge MA: Harvard University Press, 1981.

Rolf, J., Masten, A., Cicchetti, D., Nuechterlein, K., & Weintraub, S. (Eds.). *Risk and Protective Factors in the Development of Psychopathology*. Cambridge, England: Cambridge University Press, 1990.

Rudy, D.R. Slipping and sobriety: The functions of drinking in Alcoholics Anonymous. *Journal of Studies on Alcohol, 41,* 1980, 272–282.

Rutter, M. *Children of Sick Parents*. London: Oxford University Press, 1966.

Sameroff, A. J., & Seifer, R. Familial risk and child competence. *Child Development, 54,* 1983, 1254–1268.

Sameroff, A. J., Seifer, R., & Zax, M. Effects of parental emotional handicap on early child development. In S. K. Thurman (Ed.), *Children of Handicapped Parents: Research and Clinical Perspectives*. Orlando FL: Academic Press, 1985, pp. 47–66.

Sandler, J. Trauma, strain, and development. In S. S. Furst (Ed.), *Psychic Trauma*. New York: Basic Books, 1967, 154–174.

Schmid, J. Alcoholism and the family. In S. Brown (Ed.), *Treating Alcoholism*. San Francisco, Jossey-Bass, 1995, pp. 353–396.

Steinglass, P. A life history model of the alcoholic family. *Family Process, 19*(3), 1980, 211–226.

Steinglass, P., Bennett, L., Wolin, S., & Reiss, D. *The Alcoholic Family*. New York: Basic Books, 1987.

Stern, D. *The Interpersonal World of the Infant*. New York: Basic Books, 1985.

Sullivan, H. S. *The Interpersonal Theory of Psychiatry*. New York: Norton, 1953.

Terr, L. *Too Scared to Cry*. New York: Harper & Row, 1991.

Thurman, S. K. Ecological congruence in the study of families of handicapped persons. In S. K. Thurman (Ed.), *Children of Handicapped Parents: Research and Clinical Perspectives*. Orlando, FL: Academic Press, 1985, pp. 35–43.

Tiebout, H. Therapeutic mechanisms of Alcoholics Anonymous. *American Journal of Psychiatry, 100,* 1944, 468–473.

Tiebout, H. Psychological factors operating in Alcoholics Anonymous. In B. Glueck (Ed.), *Current Therapies of Personality Disorders*. New York: Grune & Stratton, 1946, pp. 145–165.

Tiebout, H. The act of surrender in the psychotherapeutic process with special reference to alcoholism. *Quarterly Journal of Studies on Alcohol, 10,* 1949, 48–58.

Tiebout, H. Surrender vs. compliance in therapy with special reference to alcoholism. *Quarterly Journal of Studies on Alcohol, 14,* 1953, 58–68.

Treadway, D. C. *Before It's Too Late: Working with Substance Abuse in the Family.* New York: Norton, 1989.

Vaillant, G. *The Natural History of Alcoholism.* Cambridge, MA: Harvard University Press, 1983.

Van Bree, G. Treating the alcoholic couple. In S. Brown (Ed.), *Treating Alcoholism.* San Francisco: Jossey-Bass, 1995, pp. 317–352.

van der Kolk, B. (Ed.). *Psychological Trauma.* Washington, DC: American Psychiatric Press, 1987.

van der Kolk, B. A., McFarlane, A. C., & Weisaeth, L. (Eds.). *Traumatic Stress.* New York: Guilford Press, 1996.

Vanicelli, M., *Group Psychotherapy with Adult Children of Alcoholics.* New York: Guilford Press, 1989.

von Bertalanffy, L. *General Systems Theory: Foundation, Development, and Applications.* New York: Braziller, 1968.

Watzlawick, P., Weakland, J., & Fisch, R. *Change.* Palo Alto, CA: Science & Behavior Books, 1974.

Webster's Third New International Dictionary of the English Language Unabridged. Springfield MA: Merriam-Webster, 1981 (originally published in 1961).

Wegsheider, S. *Another Chance: Hope and Health for the Alcoholic Family.* Palo Alto, CA: Science & Behavior Books, 1981.

Weiss, J. *How Psychotherapy Works.* New York: Guilford Press, 1993.

Weiss, J., Sampson, H., & the Mount Zion Psychotherapy Research Group. *The Psychoanalytic Process: Theory, Clinical Observations, and Empirical Research.* New York: Guilford Press, 1986.

Winnicott, D. W. Transitional objects and transitional phenomena. *International Journal of Psycho-Analysis, 34,* 1953, 89–97.

Winnicott, D. W. The theory of the parent–infant relationship. *International Journal of Psycho-Analysis, 41,* 1960, 585–595.

Winnicott, D. W. *The Maturational Processes and the Facilitating Environment.* New York: International Universities Press, 1965.

Wolin, S., & Bennett, L. Family rituals. *Family Process, 23,* 1984, 401–420.

Wolin, S., Bennett, L., & Noonan, D. Family rituals and the reoccurrence of alcoholism over generations. *American Journal of Psychiatry, 136,* 1979, 589–593.

Wolin, S., Bennett, L., Noonan, D., & Teitelbaum, M. A. Disrupted family rituals. *Journal of Studies on Alcohol, 41,* 1980, 199–214.

Wood, B. *Children of Alcoholism: The Struggle for Self and Intimacy in Adult Life.* New York: New York University Press, 1987.

Wurmser, L. *The Hidden Dimension: Psychodynamics in Compulsive Drug Use.* New York: Aronson, 1978.

Zweben, J. The therapist's role in early and ongoing recovery. In S. Brown (Ed.), *Treating Alcoholism.* San Francisco: Jossey-Bass, 1995, pp. 1197–1229.

Index

Note: Page numbers in boldface denote Glossary entries.